Do Men Like Fat Women?

By Chican C.M.V.

*To all those beautiful curvaceous
and plus-size women.*

Contents

The woman who started it all

"Too fat!" the tall boy whispered to his pal while turning his back to the women. He did not seem to be interested anymore in the women from our compartment. He sat straight ahead and started glancing out the subway window. Nothing from our compartment was interesting enough for him, not even his pals.

Thirty minutes earlier:

It all started as an ordinary morning one summer. On this particular day, my friend and I took the subway from the city outskirts to reach the center of the city, a trip of around thirty to forty minutes.

While waiting for the subway, we were intensely debating over a Norwegian movie, having different opinions about it. From time to time, some of the corporate women passing near us distracted our attention for a couple of seconds. Now, you might ask yourself why men who had a life partner were still looking at other women. Perhaps not all do it, but most I know do it. It is quite simple. They just cannot resist it. It is in the nature of many men to have their attention attracted by some women. In a TV documentary, this could be explained in a scientific yet controversial way, as if revealing the discovery of the century. The TV documentary could say that the visual appearance or scent of a woman triggers some chemical reaction in a man's brain that stimulates key...I do not know what, and so on. Nevertheless, keeping it simple, we can consider that women, because of their nature, attract many, if not most men. This does not mean that men cannot be loyal to one woman, or deeply in love or committed to their partner; is just that for many men, some things are beyond their control.

Coming back to our story, there were not so many people waiting for the subway that morning. Beside us, there were around ten well-dressed office workers, a group of young men in their early twenties, and few other people in the distance.

The subway arrived and we got into one of its compartments. There were not many people inside our compartment, and most of the seats were free. Even the air seemed to be cleaner and fresher than usual. The group of young men also entered in our compartment and sat down pretty close to us. They were making quite a lot of noise, interrupted only from time to time by the train. I remember looking at them and envying their freshness and restless enthusiasm. They were restlessly speaking, and from time to time loudly laughing. Soon the door closed and a voice announced the next station.

Because the young men near us were making so much noise, somehow it did not make any more sense for me and my friend to continue our debate about the movie. Therefore, we switched the conversation to something less contrary, mixed with moments of silence and self-reflection.

At the next stop, two people joined us in our compartment. An older man, who chose a seat close to the door, and a tall slim girl, who was pretty close the same age as the young men— probably a student. She chose a seat that was in front of the young men.

Even if the girl was dressed summery, she was quite presentable. She was dressed in brown shorts, a short pink T-shirt, and high-heel sandals. Her thin and slim body was in a very straight and impressive posture. Though she was wearing a hat, I noticed her beautiful, straight, and long blonde hair falling down her shoulders. After a few moments, she took her hat off and placed it on the empty seat near her. Just after she let go of the hat, it fell down on the compartment floor and began to roll. I was surprised to see that instead of rushing to pick it up off the floor, she slowly moved her head back and smiled with her mouth slightly open. It was as if she had a personal story with the hat and she was amused by the fact it was running from her. For a couple of seconds, her broad smile and twinkling eyes took everyone's attention in the compartment. I could not avoid noticing her thin face, small dark eyes, and thin eyebrows. While still smiling and showing her healthy teeth, she bent over and suddenly, with a smooth and open movement, took the hat from the floor and placed it on the seat near her. Once the hat was in the desired place, she did not remove her hand quickly. Instead, she kept her fingers above the hat for few more seconds. Her fingers were touching the hat in a caring way, as if the hat was a naughty pet not listening to its master. Then she crossed her legs gracefully, by placing one leg above the other one, stretching, and pressing her spotless skin together. A minute later, she put her hand to rest above her knee.

The group of young men had started to react even before she chose her seat. They were smiling, giggling, whispering, and trying to attract her attention. Some of the boys were trying to call attention to themselves more, by speaking slightly louder or by throwing long looks at the girl. Among them, one tall, dark-haired man seemed to be quite self-confident and appreciated in the group.

Even if there was a slight combativeness among them to attract the girl's attention, it seemed that the boys were feeling good and satisfied about their hesitant looks and reactions.

Initially, I thought that the girl did not notice the giggling and gestures of the group. However, the way she tossed her head and her repeated slight hand movements through her hair, together with quick evasive looks in the directions of the young men convinced me that she was quite aware of all the attention she had garnered. During this time, my friend and I were also glancing from time to time into her direction.

At the next station, another woman entered our compartment. She was around twenty-five to thirty years old and she chose a seat just at a few seats distance from the girl. Initially, the group of young men did not notice her because of their focus and interest on the tall girl.

The new woman that joined us in the compartment had a corpulent body, with obvious curvy shapes. She had freckled skin and medium-length, wavy, light brown hair. She was smartly dressed in a formal suit consisting of a dark jacket and a straight skirt of the same color, hitting just below her knees. Underneath her jacket, she had a buttoned white shirt, which was quite tight for her body; the buttons next to some areas around her waist and bust looked as if they were about to pop off. She also seemed to be aware of this, since from time to time she brought one of her hands, which were hesitantly fidgeting over her stomach, to straighten her shirt area between the buttons. She also had on classical flat shoes that fit her quite nicely.

From the moment I saw her, I noticed that, most of the time, her eyes were looking down, with slight movements from side to side. Even after she sat down, she kept her head slightly down and did not look around. Later on, I noticed her full, rounded face, sorrowful yet expressive blue eyes, and thick eyebrows.

After sitting down, her body shape and curves were even more obvious. The curves of her hips became highly pronounced and were hard not to notice. It was not long before most men from the compartment noticed her. In the beginning, it was quite hard to avoid looking into her direction. However, shortly after, perhaps not to be rude or so obvious, it was quite hard to look in her direction. In my case, most of the time, I was looking in very strange directions. At some point, I met the eyes of my friend, and instantaneously I recognized he had the same puzzled face. When we both realized that she had the same effect on us, we smiled at each other, like a silent agreement.

There was also something strange about her. On the one hand, her body curves were very attractive, sexy and appealing—in pleasant way, not vulgar. On the other hand, she seemed shy and fragile, with her body collapsed on itself and her head lowered between her slouching shoulders.

It did not take me long to notice that there was far more silence in our compartment and that the young men were saying nothing. Nothing! They were not even giggling anymore about the slim girl. All of them were standing in their places, and from time to time, they gave each other quick and tense looks in the direction of the curvaceous woman.

It was obvious she had an intense effect on us. After some time, some of the young men started a conversation in their group. However, now it was somehow different. It was as if they were trying to look more mature than they were. There was no giggling and there was more seriousness and tension in their gestures. In addition, their looks in the direction of the curvaceous woman were shorter and reserved, as if they were somehow intimidated by her or by each other in their group.

My friend and I were acting similar to the young men. Even if she was tremendously attractive, we were looking in all kinds of directions. It was as if the view in front of us was not interesting at all.

It might have been that the sexiness of her body shapes, combined with how her large curvaceous body was fitting the space, was intimidating to us. Actually, I had no idea at that moment why both of us were so reserved about looking in her direction.

At some point, I dared to take a better look, and I was able to see both women. Then the difference between them struck me. The curvaceous-shaped woman had a far more attractive body. Even more, her look was highly in contrast to the shining appearance of the thin woman. The curved position of her head, the humble position of her back, her hesitant gestures, her sad eyes looking almost continuously at the floor, contrasted the look and attitude of the tall girl. This did not make any sense to me since her curvaceous body was having a huge impact on all the men in the compartment. Perhaps not on the old man, but who knows, I did not pay attention to him at that moment.

Few moments later, her mobile phone rang and I noticed that it took her some time to take the mobile out of her bag. She finally found it, and with a very low and hesitant voice, she answered the call. After she finished her short conversation, she fiddled with her phone for few minutes, and then placed her hands back over her stomach. It crossed my mind that she might be uncomfortable because of the men gazing at her, but then I realized that compared to the thin woman, she had fewer direct looks or attention from the men in the compartment. Both the young men's group and we (my friend and I) were avoiding looking in her direction. Also, the young men were more reserved and did not whisper or giggle as they did with the tall slim girl. The tall, dark-haired boy especially surprised me with his reaction.

Introduction

First, welcome and thank you for taking your time to read our book.

We (the authors, both men) like and generally are attracted by curvaceous and plus-size women. Therefore, within the pages of this book, you may notice that we get slightly emotional or enthusiastic about some topics because of our personal preferences. Even so, we are committed to giving you a new, unique, and useful perspective on how men see curvaceous and plus-size women. We also give information and tips on how curvaceous women and plus-size women can increase their attractiveness to men.

Writing this book was not an easy thing to do. We had to spend a lot of time thinking about and discussing how it could be useful, and rephrasing and reviewing it to give you the best possible view on how men perceive curvaceous women and plus-size women and how women can be more appealing.

You might notice that we did not go too deep into some topics. We are aware of this; and this happened because we decided to focus on the key question of the book: "Why do men prefer curvy women and plus-size women?" and on topics, tips, and advice about what makes a woman more attractive to men.

After finishing this book, being afraid how women might perceive it, we asked our life partners and close female friends to read it. The feedback was positive and enthusiastic with a small exception. One friend, quite a real busybody, criticized us a lot, not agreeing with many of the ideas we expressed. We appreciated her feedback, even if she was quite a thin and slim woman—which could have something to do with her reaction. Since most of the feedback received from our other friends was surprisingly pleasant, we let it go to the publishing house; and now it has reached your hands. We hope you enjoy it!

Are curvy and plus-size women sexy and attractive?

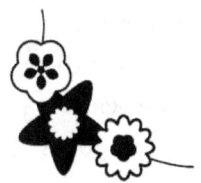

Curvy and plus size could be considered, in many cases, words that evoke the image of a real woman, suggesting naturalness and womanly forms of expression. Some might even consider them an agreement between a woman and nature, a commitment to the idea of showing and appreciating a woman's shape.. Through the promise of variety and the uniqueness of body shapes, curvy and plus-size women place us in the world of women's sensuality and beauty.

Plus size is a term widely used today, and many women who have plus-size clothing needs are not comfortable with it. This feeling could be because society is promoting certain so-called standards for women's body size and shape, in which plus size does not fir. Many women consider the standard model promoted by society as the ideal model of beauty. Furthermore, they see it as the path to success, fulfillment, and social achievement. Because of these beliefs, it is not hard to understand why they try to meet these standards and the natural response of obedience to them. This so-called ideal standard generates desires, and imposes constrains and rigors. As a result, it creates frustration, even among the most beautiful women. The ideal beauty model has a seductive character. After claiming its position in the mind of a person, it will offer, in return, frustrations, and sometimes unhappiness.

You do not have to fit society's beauty standard to be successfully in life. Any woman, no matter her look or body, can be a candidate for happiness and achieve personal fulfillment.

Curvaceous body forms show the naturalness of women. Women have all kind of shapes and sizes and they should be able to display their body without feeling bad their natural body curves, voluptuousness, or bolder forms. A well-tailored skirt or a dress carefully chosen could improve the appearance of a woman, no matter if she is thin or fat. More or less, curvaceous women's forms are a delight for the eye of many men. The curves of many plus-size women, their body voluptuousness, and the health expression in their cheeks could compete, with success, against many slim women.

Men instinctively, in most cases, will feel attracted by women regardless of their type. As long as women will suggest their availability, no matter their body shapes, they will have a very good chance of attracting the interest of men.

The awareness of many women about their body uniqueness is an important aspect. What a woman sees when she looks herself in the mirror is the most precious thing in her possession. That body serves as her reliable ally. She should not see it as an enemy or a target for all kinds of diets because she wants to meet a standard. Of course, that body has a different shape than other women. It might have a different weight, a different size of the hips or breasts. All of these differences give more character to the body and makes it particularly memorable for a man. If something matters most when it comes to the female body, it is that difference. You should not measure the beauty of a woman in kilograms or pounds, centimeters or inches, or depending on skin, hair, or eye color.

Does it make sense that only a certain kind of woman could be attractive? Attractiveness and sexiness are specific attributes to all women, regardless of race, social class, skin color, sexual orientation, or religion. Of course, at a specific moment, a woman could be less or more attractive than another. Even so, considering the variety of people who give an opinion about a woman, subjectivity may be the only certainty.

To provide a ranking evaluation commonly requires a system by which to evaluate. That system will enforce standards. In addition, it will have some precise measuring instruments, and some principles to follow. It will also require people to believe and embrace its meanings, and people to use it. As long as evaluations focus on rational things, these systems will serve their purpose. Still, when it comes to women's attractiveness, it is almost impossible to draw up such a credible system. To consider a woman attractive is a subjective matter. The eyes see images and the human brain assigns specific meanings to them. The education, social life, emotional life, and experiences of a specific person influence the significance of these meanings.

From one point of view or from a particular perspective, a woman could be very attractive. Yet, this fact cannot be a general valid truth, since it is quite subjective, emotional, and personal. Attractiveness of a woman is more a thing bound to feelings and less to the judgment of mind. Attractiveness could be a language that speaks to the heart and impresses the soul. Therefore, the brain may be unable to interpret these signals consciously. Each of us perceives attractiveness differently, because each of us feels things differently. When it is about attractiveness, we desert the rational area and the emotional area takes the lead. In this respect, things tend to manifest more complex and illogical judgments and analytical thinking tends to lose validity.

Is a curvy and plus-size woman attractive enough? There is no satisfactory and easy answer to this question. Attractiveness may be physical if we consider the person's unique physical traits. However, attractiveness can be of a psychological nature, especially when there are similarities in the way of thinking. The key of attractiveness, therefore, could be highlighting the value of specific physical or psychological aspects that might make a particular woman shine. Any woman could be attractive, because every woman has a special charm. An important thing for women who desire to be more attractive is to be aware of their unique aspects and their own ability to emphasize them. It is quite hard to imagine a woman who could not generate interest or desire. Most women could attract attention or seduce almost instinctively, as long as they are aware of their key strengths and know how to exploit them.

A woman could be wonderful. She could create another world with just a kind word, a hug, or a kiss. Still, many women forget this every time after doing it.

Beauty, sex appeal, and attractiveness

Beauty

We cannot talk about a woman, without referring to her beauty. Women are beautiful by definition. Feminine beauty has inspired artists from all centuries. Each of them sang, painted, or wrote beauty as they felt it. Artists defined and presented the beauty in their artwork according to their times. In public, many artists presented their vision of ideal beauty, and from their creations, we can see their concept come to life. However, beauty has been defined through the centuries on volatile attributes, sensitive to the passage of time and changing attitudes.

The beauty of full-figured Rubenesque women has a set of attributes that are in high contrasting with many current perceptions about beauty. Beauty seems to be a subjective and changing. Therefore, identifying the attributes of feminine beauty was and will be an intense interest of human society.

In a large sense, women's beauty derives from the broad variety of feminine forms and of their peculiarities. It is impossible to find two identical women with the same body. Beauty can take varied forms. Moreover, if we consider the variety of races, we will come to understand how complex and divers the manifestation of beauty is. Each race could suggest an ideal model of beauty based on specific traits to that race. Some might even propose several such models as ideal. It is about the shape of the eyes, nose, lips, cheek, skin, hair, body stature, and other specific features that female beauty and variety will manifest in all itself splendor. Nevertheless, the differences between these beauty ideals add to the subjectivity of defining one beauty ideal, as they have obvious differences between them.

The problem in defining a beauty ideal is that it is hard to find non-subjective criteria for evaluating beauty. A measurement instrument used for detecting the beauty of one race may be at the expense of others. Who will advise such a tool—this subjective manifestation of human society in its quest to find beautiful women?

Beauty is universal. We can admire it in every woman. It has existed and will exist all around us, even if we are able to identify only the beauty suggested by others. Each mother, sister, wife, girlfriend, or daughter is suspected at one time to be the most beautiful woman in her universe. Thus, every woman gets to mirror her beauty in the eyes of someone like her son, brother, husband, boyfriend, or father.

However, often we identify beauty where nobody seems to see that it exists. It could also happen that what some might find just ordinary, others could identify as extraordinarily beautiful. The factors or filters specific to each individual, such as education, social status, and their own system of values or personal convictions influence the perception of beauty.

Nowadays, society promotes more or less faulty notions of beauty ideals, so you do not have to meet exactly these ideals for being beautiful. It should be each woman's responsibility to assess her own body in terms of features and uniqueness without necessarily relating to specific social standards.

Beauty can be an abstract term. Some might say it's an asset; others might consider it an attribute, a quality, or a subjective evaluation. Identifying the definition and meaning of beauty was the concern of many of our peers. Along time ago, many famous personalities, such as Oscar Wilde, Francis Bacon, Confucius, William Shakespeare, Plato, Aristotle, and Immanuel Kant appreciated beauty and aesthetics in their own way and vision.

In addition to physical aesthetics, you can see the inner beauty of a person. Inner beauty of the soul is a different dimension, and often neglected by people. Even so, this dimension tends to be as important, if not more important, as outer beauty. This little-publicized area of beauty has several advantages, and has much to give to humankind. The inner side of beauty is the one that can be preserved or ever blossom over time. Together with age, inner beauty has a chance to increase and to improve.

Unfortunately, we cannot say that outer physical beauty preserves also over time.

Nowadays, more and more people tend to put value on the purely physical aspects of their peers. Nevertheless, it seems that physical aspects are not enough when it comes to developing and maintain long lasting healthy relationships. In the case of great and excellent relationships, outer beauty can only be complementary to spiritual/inner beauty. In many cases, outer appearance draws the attention of a man and triggers the beginning of a relationship. However, when it comes to the quality, intensity, and longevity of a relationship, inner beauty plays a key role. Inner beauty provides proper soil for cultivation of long lasting relationships.

Some might consider that women are more skillful at identifying the richness of the human soul. In addition, they know about appreciating this hidden beauty.

Men tend, instead, to focus in the area of alluring seductive female body shapes. An early voyage into the woman's soul might not be handy for many men. For younger men, it is even harder not to have their eyes engaged in the lure of femininity. Therefore, in many cases, men fail to penetrate the inner beauty of women's soul in the beginning of a relationship.

An important factor to consider while speaking about beauty is the health. Health might contribute to the overall beauty of person, or at least to how she sees herself. Health is the state in which the human body functions optimally. To have a body functioning within normal parameters, an important aspect might be focusing on one's daily lifestyle. For example, a balanced diet could contribute to the health of a person. Daily adequate physical exercises, resting moments, and avoiding excesses also contribute to one's health. In addition, it is quite important, if you have been or might be susceptible to serious health problems, to ask for help and advice on possible approaches from a professional.

Sex appeal and attractiveness

Sex appeal involves a physical personal quality of a woman that gives her a sort of arousing charm and unique attractiveness in comparison to others. When the sex appeal of a woman is powerful, feelings of admiration or even jealousy could appear around her. Many women might have feelings of jealousy when it is obvious that some men think that she has more sex appeal. You should keep in mind that every woman has her personal charm. A woman could use these charms to her advantage and for standing out. By using her personal charms, a woman could increase her chances of attracting men. In other words, we could say that sex appeal is based on attraction between the partners.

Success commonly belongs to those women who have acquired skills to highlight the features that make them shine. In many cases, men will appreciate more the women who are conscious of their particular key strengths and have the ability to expose these key personal qualities in a favorable manner.

A woman's ability to arouse desire or interest in men could be the foundation of attraction. Commonly, many people feel an attraction toward those who are as attractive or as intelligent as they are. Even so, it is also quite common for men to be attracted by opposite qualities. For example, many men with thin lips like women with thick lips.

Attractiveness may depend, in many cases, on proximity. Proximity is a key factor in the possibility of interactions. The closer you are, the more you interact and the more chances for attraction. By interacting more often, people will become aware of their common interests or passions. Similar interests could increase attraction in many cases. It is quite common for people who share interests, passions, or hobbies to feel a strong attraction for each other. For many, it is more comfortable to interact with people who have the same attitude or share the same values. Furthermore, is quite common for men to like women who are more agreeable and show an active genuine interest in them.

Physical attractiveness may be manifested both at the face and body level. Some believe facial attractiveness plays a more important role than body attractiveness, while others believe the opposite. In many cases, the face of a woman gives the first impression of beauty. The beauty of the eyes, their expression, the thickness and movement of their lips are some of the first elements that create an impression during a discussion. After focusing on facial aspects, many men will shift their attention to the body, for an overall view of the woman. Key parts of the body carefully exposed, together with a smart outfit and accessories, could attract a man's attention even more. Even so, facial attractiveness is still key for the overall attractiveness of a woman.

You should not ignore the fact that the power to attract and maintain attention is in almost every woman at specific times. In many cases, when a woman looks more attractive, it is only because she knows how to add value in a tactfully manner to her key or unique characteristics. For maximizing her attractiveness, a woman will have to be aware and confident of her unique key points.

Sometimes even defects could contribute to a woman's image and attractiveness. In other cases, perfect symmetry could often fool the eye as an enjoyable, pleasant, and attractive image. Additionally, with adequate self-confidence and a confident approach, positive perception of physical appearance could happen even where nature has not been very generous.

In other words, while physical appearance is important in the attraction between people and makes the difference in the first phase of a relationship, elements like character or temperament could become more important later.

Generally, we evaluate physical appearance, which we can see and explore with the eye. Often we appreciate a neat appearance, the quality of clothes, a color, and even gestures or mannerisms of a person. Many men are true aesthetic detectors. However, a woman could reach the maximum attractiveness potential when, beside her beautiful appearance, she shows her inner beauty, self-esteem, and self-confidence. The appreciation of others can often influence personal fulfillment and satisfaction. Appreciation from those who represent our personal world has a huge effect on our feelings of accomplishment. The opinions of others affect us less if we have a strong feeling of fulfillment, self-confidence, and personal accomplishment. Somehow, this creates a paradox, since it is harder to reach this state without being powered by others' appreciations.

A brief history of what men find attractive

People have been and will always be concerned about beauty. Women are definitely more concerned about appearance and about how they look. In many cases, if not most of them, men will respond positively to women who carefully and skillfully show their beauty. Skillfully displaying certain physical traits could empower many women to engage men's attention, as women's beauty has been able to captivate the hearts of men for centuries.

During the last centuries, the so-called standards of beauty have changed many times. Furthermore, they will continue to change in the future. Present and future developments in science and technology, in areas such as cyberspace, genetics, and virtual reality could offer new dimensions of beauty, and endless possibilities. Ideas that might sound wild now, like replacing or drastically changing your physical appearance could be a possibility in the not so distant future. Perhaps there will be women who would borrow the unique features of Aphrodite or other celebrities.

Long ago, men probably felt attracted to the physical beauty of someone like Eve, the inner beauty of Mary, or the irresistible beauty of the Italian Renaissance Gioconda. They loved and adored these women, and together they created families. Men will love women for what they are, as long as humanity exists.

Praxiteles, a well-known sculptor of Athens, showed a woman with a well-proportioned body, mature breasts, and full hips in beauty of "Aphrodite". This work of art is widely known as one of the first nude artworks in classical sculpture. With the help of a hammer and a chisel, he was able to carve in rock the faithful representation of the perfect woman's body of those times.

Later, during the Italian Renaissance we can find an abundance of representations of women's beauty. An artwork focusing on the feminine forms is the "Birth of Venus", created by Sandro Botticelli. This masterpiece was built at the command of Lorenzo and Giovanni di Pierfrancesco de Medici, some of the most wealthy and influential families in Italy at that time.

Annibale Carracci, an outstanding representative of Renaissance period, is also one of the artists who found inspirations in the traditional form of women's beauty. Within his artwork, we can find influences of the ancient Greek goddess Venus.

The renaissance painter Guido Canlassi, insisted on showing the beautiful seductive forms of his time in his works. His sensual artwork "The Death of Cleopatra" shows the curvaceous beauty of those times.

As a contemporary of Leonardo Da Vinci, Giampietrino described in his artwork Lukretia, the woman with round breasts, a robust body, and bright red hair. Many representatives of the Renaissance era shared his vision of female beauty. Pieter Paul Rubens also devoted his attention and life to creating beautiful representations of curvaceous, robust women's bodies. Even Rembrandt honors women's bodies in his work.

These various art works dedicated to beauty support the idea of a variety and complexity of forms that define beauty. This is proof that beauty can have variety, even the uniqueness, in the shapes or lines of women body.

Who can better represent the emotions generated by the female body form if not artists? Their works speak without words to the feelings they had about women's beauty. In addition, their works shows sublime admiration for various types and body shapes.

Maybe other women from our past wanted to get closer to the ideal of beauty specific to their time. On the other hand, maybe they did not feel the pressure of a beauty model as many women do today. They definitely did not feel the pressure of a powerful mass media, as the one from our time. Many might say that media, like radio, television, newspapers, magazines, and the Internet seed the mind with various models and standards of beauty, and that those models can only be ephemeral.

Could the physical beauties from the art works of Leonardo Da Vinci, Edouard Manet, and Peter Paul Rubens compete with today's beauty models? How would we feel about those muses of inspiration if they could time travel to our contemporary society? Would we appreciate their beauty as it was in their time?

Today, the beauty models of our society are not just gimmicks designed to create random frustration or happiness among women. Real examples of successful women and men stimulate and motivate many to adopt these models; they accept the rules of the game. The winners of the beauty game will take the laurels, while the losers will mostly have frustrations. Such frustrations could often lead to anger or fear. In this context, it is the fear of exclusion, marginalization. It also might be the fear of others ignoring or not noticing you. Fear is natural. It was responsible for our preservation as a species throughout the centuries. Without fear, women and men would have perished a long time ago.

Nevertheless, in our case, fear is artificial. Many ideal qualities of existing beauty models could be false, and some might be used to discourage and create complexes for most women. An underlying issue could be interests that have far less to do with beauty or appreciation of women.

What is natural?

The natural aspect of women's beauty could be in the diversity and uniqueness of forms. Attempts to measure this naturalness or beauty by assigning it to a specific standard might result in reducing beauty to trivial aspects of it. Focusing too much on the compliance with some beauty standard might give birth to discomfort or frustration among specific people. In extreme scenarios, it even might give birth to racism.

In today's society, many create and promote ideal beauty models with the purpose of gaining people's attention. These models generate desires and deviate attention from other critical societal themes. How many women buy a cosmetic product for the product itself? What is the necessity for a lipstick or eyeliner? Are women buying the illusion that using these products will make them more beautiful or more easily noticed in their environment? In this way, some might exploit weaknesses and encourage vanity. By exploiting human weaknesses, the need to feel beautiful and noticed, specific key players benefit greatly. A society that creates, promotes, and exploits human weaknesses may wake up one day poorer as a result.

Implantation, injections, and adding or removing certain parts of the human body is a practice commonly used today. Of course, there might be cases where such interventions are driven by real health necessities and have nothing to do with so-called beauty model compliance. However, in many cases, some actions that target the woman's body defy the natural and violates body integrity. Still, many women are doing it because they want to comply with certain beauty models and need more recognition and admiration from society. Many businesses promote successful stories of those who have already resorted to such additions or eliminations. They emphasize that after surgery, the woman suddenly increased her confidence and self-esteem. Miraculously her life changed and everything that seemed dark became light.

However, any change, even if it seems to come from the outside, is only an impression; it is just an illusion. The real change always comes from within. Nevertheless, it is easier to believe that upon them with different. Actually, in most cases, we do not need such interventions to enjoy the appreciation of the people surrounding us. As long as we focus on our key strengths and not weaknesses, we look confident to the world. We shouldn't consider certain traits as weaknesses just because the society in which we live suggests it. Perhaps in other societies those traits would be an advantage. The moral duty of our society should be to cultivate a positive attitude. We should be educated to appreciate the way we look and not how we *should* look. To love ourselves for what we are, not for what we *could be.*

Some might say that in some turbulent periods in history, only those women belonging to dominant groups of that time met the ideals of beauty. Today, dominant organizations and corporations on consumer goods market heavily to promote their visions of women beauty ideals. In their search for a bigger market share, these corporations are able to impress by promoting the so-called perfect models of beauty. Then they will suggest that just by using their product you could reach that ideal. In this way, they create the illusion that the consumption of their products will allow individual fulfillment. By designing and promoting a strict and hard to achieve beauty standard, they aim intentionally at mass frustration. The greater the number of people who do not meet the standard and who feel frustration, the greater product sales.

We cannot standardize the complexity or diversity of female beauty. Standards are not able to include the sublime feminine beauty of every woman. Standards could only be a moment of improvisation, an abstract tool, an artificial representation of beauty. Such instruments cannot measure women's beauty. An industry could support a standard for a product, and many times, it really needs it. By using standards, various industries could achieve the optimization of quality. However, a woman is born beautiful and will not need to undergo a whole process of standardization in order to demonstrate this quality. She is not a consumer product but a unique human being. Therefore, a woman is superior to any standard made by man. Even so, we could compare a woman with another one. Nevertheless, the conclusion can only be subjective. It will reflect only a specific point of view and reveal impressions of specific benchmarks under the influence of culture, education, or the social environment of the individual who judges it.

It is obvious in our society that there is an interest and tendency to standardize the woman beauty. If a woman is the manifestation of nature, trying to standardize her beauty may be similar to trying to create standard landscapes around us. Could you imagine the same landscape all around you, from north to south and from east to west? If this happened, most probably we would greatly admire any variation that broke the monotony. Could we ever consider that the oak tree forests is obsolete as a beauty standard and to try to replace it all with something exotic like palm trees just because they are in trend now?

By its variety, nature itself is beauty. Moreover, we cannot limit its beauty by any standard created by man. Man has always been tempted to reduce complexity. Thus, it is easier to him to generate certain meanings in order to serve his own interest. Standardization in this sense is a measure capable of meeting specific human purposes.

Maybe we should ask ourselves why the separation from a love partner affects us, considering that there are millions of women and men around us. Is not her or his uniqueness the thing that we really miss? Is not the uniqueness the one responsible for a strong bond? So, why do we need to have or to impose beauty standards? Instead, difference itself is what could be a standard. Each woman has a specific meaning in her relationships with men. Men should love a woman for what she is and means to them, not for her closeness to a model suggested by one industry or another. However, many men already do this.

Beauty is wild and we cannot frame it into a standard. Only someone naive could believe that we can keep beauty a standard. Because of their need and desire of societal appreciation, many women are subjects of the ideal beauty models made by society, ignoring the fact that they already represent beauty in this world.

Attention and importance

If men would admire and desire only one type of women, competition between men could reach huge dimensions. Such a model, frequently promoted, might narrow the horizon of individuals and make them ignore their options. Even so, advertising and marketing is pushing various beauty standards ahead. After the elite and trendsetters adopt a particular standard, many, if not most, will adopt it also. Therefore, an ally in promoting the ideal beauty model is the very nature of man and his ability to imitate others. Few will be those who will depart from the trend, perhaps because of fear for their exclusion.

Diversity could mean harmony. The fact that everyone is different, feels different, and behaves differently creates alternatives to others. Standardization could cancel the variety, support alienation, and damage harmony.

In many scenarios today, society distorts reality by suggesting that compliance with a beauty standard is an ideal of social achievement. Under the dictatorship of commercial advertising, the body seems to become a fashion accessory. Day by day, aggressive advertising promotes ideal models of beauty. However, the ongoing effort to conform to these beauty or fashion standard and trends will generate and increase frustration among many.

Most people tend to avoid responsibility for their decisions. This weakness was always quite common among people. They feel safer letting others make decisions for them. Even if they never clearly express their expectations or interests, they imagine that those who are making the decisions will consider their wishes and interests.

The same happens when it comes to beauty and ideal models. Since it is far easier to have some guidelines, we could consider that many people are asking for models. Many people feel it's hard to make important choices alone. The fear of being ridiculed or rejected by others causes them to choose standards widely used. Therefore, it is no surprise that many are happy when standard choices are available around us. It might be convenient to have choices on how to live, what clothes to buy, what car to buy, or what kind of hairstyle to adopt. People prefer models to remove uncertainty. Even so, the standards will not help too much when fighting against anonymity or trying to be more special. People, especially teens, try to stand out in a crowd. Because of their desire to attract attention from us, we intentionally wear dull clothes, strange haircuts, or adopt all sorts of jargon in our speech. Most of us attempt by our own means to impress others.

On the other hand, many might ridicules, exclude, or marginalize people who deviate too much from existing standards. Fear of failure inhibits many from making decisions that might make them live by their own standards. Few will have the courage to come forward and make their own choices and decisions. Moreover, many, from the ones who come forward become our models of successful women.

Successful curvy and plus-size women stories

As you might already know, many curvy women and plus-size women proved to be successfully in their personal life or career. If you are having doubts that curvy and plus-size women can be successful, go on with this chapter. Otherwise, you could skip to the next one.

Sample cases where we could see successful plus-size women:

- Society. You could simply pay a visit to a museum of history or art, such as Louvre for example. You will not have to go to France for this, there should be exhibitions in places near you, or you could just search the Internet. There you will see that many plus-size women had

an important role in society or history,
or they have been chosen as muses by
some of the greatest painters or
sculptors the world has had.

- Family. If for you family and children
play a key role in defining a successful
woman, you can find your examples by
simply visiting a beach. This beach
should not be one dedicated for
teenagers, but rather a general beach
where you can commonly find families
with children. There should be many
beaches to choose from, closer or farther
away, for example, the beautiful beaches
of Tenerife, Canary Islands. Here you
will have the occasion to see for yourself
many curvy and plus-size women who
have a great and happy family. By
looking at it, it might seem almost too
simple to achieve.

- Career. If you are considering career
advancement as a key factor to succeed
in life, there might be some areas where
it could be harder, if not almost
impossible, for some plus-size women to
build a career. However, the more we,

the authors, thought and researched this, the more we became convinced that many plus-size women could develop a successful career in most fields. The key to success, the ingredients in career advancement, might be far more focused on factors such as character, competence, work experience, soft skills, education, self-confidence, perseverance, and persuasion.

- Leadership. Leadership is not about the shape of your body. Other factors help you to evolve as a great leader. These are factors such as listening to the people, the ability to solve challenging situations, responsibility, vision, courage, competence, continuous learning, character strength, positivism, coaching, and so on.
- Superstar. Well, how about superstars? Are any of your favorites TV shows personalities curvy and plus size? There were enough examples in the TV shows that I watched this week.
- Modeling. Because modeling agencies have restrictive requirements, could a

plus-size woman still have a career in modeling? How big are your chances as a plus-size woman to appear in fashion shows, advertising campaigns, magazine editorials, catwalk work, TV commercials, stock photography, garment ads, fashion editorials, calendars, and cosmetics advertising photos, and so on? First, you should know that modeling is a tough world for all kinds of women. Even if there are modeling agencies that are searching for plus-size models, the requirements are quite tough, and even if you meet them, nobody could guarantee success. The modeling world was and will be a hard, if not impossible, target for many women, no matter if they are plus size or not. Currently, many clothing creators and fashion designers are starting to pay a lot more attention to the plus-size market, since they recognized industry potential. Therefore, they are starting to use plus-sized models in their fashion shows and events. I have the feeling that even more changes will occur in this area in the future.

The world is full of successful plus-size women as examples. If everyone starts to see the beauty in larger women, it may have some striking results. This also makes sense because as women age, they tend to be heavier.

There are many examples in many areas. Just pick an area and you will find appealing women; do a little research on the Internet if you are still not convinced.

Do plus-size women have sex appeal?

"Sex appeal" refers to a woman's charm and power of attraction. By their nature, most women in various scenarios are capable of such an attribute. It is incorrect to think that some women have sex appeal and others not. However, in reality, a woman's attractiveness could depend on how she highlights and exploits her traits. One of the key factors for getting the attention is to be self-aware about those traits that could make a woman shine. Therefore, the power to attract or to seduce should be in almost every woman, no matter her stature, body shape, skin, or hair color. There might be exceptions, but generally, it is in the nature of women to attract men.

Men's preferences vary from man to man. Men are under the influence of many factors, such as the time and place they live, their hobbies or preferences, their lifestyle, and previous life experience. Cultural and educational background also plays a key role in defining individual preferences. As an example, some Middle Eastern countries require women to cover most of their body in garments. This is quite different from most Western countries, where women dress far more openly. This comparison does not say one tradition is better than the other, it just emphasizes that men's preferences and perception differ based on their culture, location, education, and background.

Female bodies are so different that it is hard to imagine two identical body shapes, with exactly the same waists, hips, faces, and so on. It is hard to contradict nature by suggesting that certain sizes, shapes, measurements, or curves are not in the right place. Even so, some might consider that a few aspects do not fit their vision. Nevertheless, why should a particular view be above the manifestation of nature? Perfection does not consist of reaching certain ephemeral standards dictated by various industries. We should rather see perfection in the complexity of natural forms.

Men, like the women, are unique beings. Even if they share similarities, they are different. Each of them feels and sees the world in his or her unique way. Therefore, different women will attract and seduce different men in various ways, in all kind of possible scenarios and moments.

It is difficult and unrealistic to imagine the consequences of a scenario where only one type of woman is able to attract and seduce men, by using only a specific way, and at only a certain moment during her life.

Do men prefer curvy and plus size?

Women instinctively attract most men. It could be because of a magical chemistry, or the way they look. For some men, body shapes might have a higher relevance, while for other men, facial features might be a key driver. However, both the body and the face might contribute to the way a man perceives a woman. A woman's face is as important as her body to create an impression. Evaluation of facial features is also subjective, like in the case of the evaluation of a woman's body.

It is hard to image an objective evaluation of the human beauty and its physical traits because the evaluation is tied to an emotional response. Perhaps unaware, the emotional side of many men continuously evaluates women's beauty. Some individuals will appreciate some specific woman's facial traits because they reflect his notion about beauty. Such a preference or opinion may or may not coincide with another. Could we consider the face of a woman less attractive because what one man felt at some point? Most probably there are lots of opposing views and perceptions about the same person, depending on the time, place, and circumstances.

The faces of many women exhibit attractiveness. This could be because of those unique traits that provide an advantage to her. In some cases, it could be the eyes, their shape, color, or expression. In other cases, the shape or size of her nose, or the form and thickness of her lips may create a positive impression on various men. Many men and women also appreciate inner beauty. Some consider that if you are beautiful inside you are also beautiful outside.

Because of the differences between people, it is impossible to identify a universal favorite type of woman. As long as people are different, they will express different preferences. Some will probably lean toward women with large eyes and pronounced forms while other might prefer thin women with prominent breasts. Some might appreciate more those women with curly hair or those with freckles. Others will feel attracted to those women with a positive attitude. Some men might appreciate those women who look like their mothers. Common interest, hobbies, or even the work environment might make some men to fall in love with some women. There are many scenarios and possibilities for all kind of men to admire, desire, or fall in love with all kinds of women. Many men will prefer those women with whom they interact every day; in this case, proximity will play a key role in defining their preferences. Cultural, educational, or social factors can also influence a man's affinity for a specific type of women. The taste for certain traits or types is also the result of life experience. Even an individual's childhood experiences and memories could contribute to the way he perceives women as an adult. Sometimes a mother's friends can become models for which the future adult might have affinities. In other cases, mothers could contribute to shape her son's favorite type of women. However, it is hard to affirm that a woman belongs to a particular "type," as many women share common attributes and traits. It might be that various men see the same woman differently. Some of these men might find her to fit a particular type, which is pleasing and attractive for them, while others might find her uninteresting. In other words, men might see and feel an opposite level of attraction while looking at a woman because of their unique perspective. Commonly, men see what they want and what interests them. Therefore, men prefer all kinds of women. As long as men's ways of perception are different and unique, because of the uniqueness of each man, men will desire and love all kinds of women. The chances of a woman to be preferred are also benefited from the natural ability of most men to transfer their admiration from one type of women to another.

Every man will see a woman in his own way. Because any woman can be seen in various and different ways by men, any woman could be, at some point, the favorite and preferred choice of a man.

Do men like curvy women and plus-size women?

Arguably, women's forms define the world of beauty. When we are speaking about material things, form plays a key role. When something we are deciding to buy seems qualitatively similar to another thing, only the form and sometimes the price may differ. Thus, form is complex and loyal to societal trends. Sometimes form is even able to tilt the balance in our lives. Form, many times, inspires and calls one to action. In addition, it may please the eye and induce positive behaviors. For example, the automotive industry can offer us various models, which from a technical perspective may have almost the same performance. Nevertheless, in many cases, the form is the one that brings delight to the eyes of the buyer.

Of course, brand is a very important factor, but even under a dedicated name, we cannot neglect the form. Most of the well-known brands are aware of the significance of form. Many brands of products compete and try to avoid obsolete or outdated forms. Today, quality has become an obvious and normal condition for many products and brands. Because of the important need to differentiate products, many producers are focusing on the product shape. It seems that nobody intends to neglect this aspect because it seems to have become mandatory for many successful commercial approaches. Shape is a key aspect, which influences desirability and buying decisions for many products. Whether we talk about cool phones, shoes, furniture, household items, or cars, all are subject to influences of shape.

In a world dedicated to form, it will not seem abnormal that some industries try to impose ideals of shape for the feminine body. However, it is hard to see these cases as normal. The beauty created by man will never equal the beauty created by nature. We cannot see women as a commercial product and we cannot label their body shape as a commercial feature. Such an assessment is meaningless in the case of women. Women's body forms, shapes, and curves are superior by their nature to whatever commercially imposed standards exist. In the case of women, the beauty of form arises from diversity and uniqueness. In the case of commercial products, innovation makes the shape of many products shine, but the designer will hardly be able to meet the beauty from nature.

Before the creation of a product, a designer imagines the ideal form of that product. In most cases, this could not happen for the woman's body. Even so, a woman's lifestyle, actions, and decisions could influence how her body develops. Many are trying to approach the beauty of a woman's body commercially and condition it by the use of specific products or services. Major commercial corporations are creating, proposing, and promoting various models and ideals of feminine beauty. By accepting, reporting, and comparing themselves with these commercial beauty standards, women consent to the game of commercially conditioned women's beauty. Treatment of women's beauty in a commercial way does not honor, in many cases, the natural beauty uniqueness that women already possess.

The body form of a woman has always attracted men. Forms of curvy, "plus size," normal, thin, fat, less fat, tall, or short women all make men excited. Physical attraction strongly relates to the shape and form or a woman. In addition, the uniqueness of our physical traits differentiates us, and at the same time, allows us to share common traits, such as the color of eyes or hair. Feminine forms are generators of passion. They are the strong drivers of imagination and inspiration. Rivers of ink have flowed in an attempt to cover the beauty of feminine forms. Poets and writers have tried to capture its appearance in their own vision or perception.

Men's attraction cannot be limited to a single form or shape. It is almost impossible to say that only one specific shape attracts men. To identify themselves with only one form, men have to ignore the rest. This is hardly possible. Some might say this is almost impossible because many men generally react to most of the female forms.

It is interesting to notice also a woman's body shape transformation over time. For example, in the case of mature women, their body has the capacity to change its shape when it is pregnant. In addition, a woman's body size and shape could differ in different stages in her life. The laws of nature freely manifest and influence the look of the body. At various stages, the form and shape of a woman's body could be dependent on various aesthetic social perceptions. For example, an adolescent female's body might have the power to transmit energy and innocence, while the body of a mother could suggest safety, reliability, and balance. Every day we look with the same eyes, but in different ways, at the women next to us. We can look to her as our girlfriend, as the mother of our children, as a friend, or as a wife. Lust, respect, love, affection, or admiration may be various manifestations for the same women. Thus, she is able to conjure various moods, feelings, or experiences at various moments and stages of her life.

Naturalness, uniqueness, and diversity are at the base of perfection. Nature has always known to interpret beauty through shape. Through forms and shapes, nature contributes to the attraction between men and women. The ingenuousness of nature is responsible for a wide diversity of forms, shapes, tastes, and preferences.

Pronounced forms attract the attention of many men. It motivates their eyes movement toward exploration. Beyond curiosity, we find desire, admiration, and pleasure in this gesture of contemplation of a woman's voluptuousness. Naturally, the eyes of many men will watch most forms of female body shapes with interest. Sharp curves and large hips as an expression of maturity attract and tempt many men, just like other body forms' manifestations. Almost all women could enjoy the same attention from various men, regardless of her body shape, breast size, waist size, or whatever her stature.

It is quite common that people tend to consider one aesthetic over another, or label a woman as more beautiful than another. Nevertheless, does beauty need comparison? What happens if two men consider various women as the *most* beautiful? Is any of them right? Should one change his opinion because the other ones promote arguments better for their preference? Humanity might still be unable to identify and be aware of all its beauties. Each century had its candidates to various beauty ideals and many women want to identify themselves with these beauty ideals. Maybe the solution for the identification and appreciation of women's beauty is not comparison.

Could we consider that true beauty has a guaranteed period of one year, two years or more? In our world, there are cases when we designate, according to specific standards, a woman as the most beautiful woman of our planet only for one year. Then we repeat the process and another woman takes her place as the most beautiful woman of our planet. Some might assume that beauty is a big effort and she can wear it for only one year. We were educated to respect certain rules in childhood. This game of beauty has its rules and standards. Still, it seems that many can change these rules at will. Each year, during various beauty contests, competitions, or evaluations, new subjective beauty preferences materialize. However, is this really about beauty? Depending on when and where you are or have been, "beautiful" might become a word without meaning in a world where many people have long forgotten what beauty really means. On the other hand, perhaps the game, competitions, and discussions about beauty are more important to us than beauty itself.

Many people look to others, waiting for them to invent beauty in order to enjoy it. Some act as if they are unable to enjoy or see beauty without a little help, guidance, or approval. Big companies are exploiting these weaknesses commercially by suggesting various models of beauty. The continuous exposure to commercially bright packages, sensational and trendy beauty concepts, make many become unable to see or admire the surrounding natural beauty. It is hard not to notice that many ways of feminine beauty contemplation are also sources of profits. Into a world where we focus on consumption and substantial gains, the search and appreciation of beauty might be less natural. Even so, against the aggressive promotion of various beauty models, it is in the nature of most men to appreciate various manifestations of woman's beauty.

What do men want?

Generally, men feel attracted to women just as women are attracted to men. Nothing is different in this regard. This primary instinct drives most of us. The procreation instinct drives the interaction between men and women. Even if there are big differences between us, we commonly try to find and choose a partner that will suit us better. In this sense, various natural, social, or cultural similarities might have an important role.

Men have different tastes and preferences about women. Physical, mental, or cultural differences between people may be the source of their different tastes. Therefore, many men will prefer curvy or plus-size women, but also many men will prefer thin women. It is worth noticing that not all men see or think the same. A man or a group of men might see a woman as normal sized, curvy, fat, or thin, while other men might see and consider her differently.

The diversity in men's tastes and preferences bring more harmony and balance to our society. The desire to meet their dream woman, to find their dream partner, drives most men. Some men might have in their mind only one model of an ideal woman, ignoring any other options around them. What would happen to other women who cannot fit this ideal model? Should they expect that new generations of men might have a new ideal woman that will include them? Actually, this is not as big an issue as it might seem. Even if some men might have a very clear idea of what kind of women they are searching for, most of them will not stick to this idea for their entire life. There are also far more men flexible and open to various options. In addition, no human society can impose only one kind of woman as desirable. As long as there is diversity, people can enjoy each other. Diversity brings happiness both to women and men. It also gives each of us more chances and choices. It is in the nature of men to react differently to various women, in this way preserving an overall balance.

From an intimate perspective, it is not in the nature of men to search for only a certain kind of woman. This means, that there is no predetermined pattern and men could act in various ways based on their character, values, life experience, and culture. Many men, especially young ones, will be quite open to variety and open to various opportunities.

It is hard to imagine men sticking to a single physical model. It is physically impossible for most men to identify and search for only a certain model. It is hard to imagine a society where all men have clear requirements or standards about stature, breast shape, waist size, weight, hair color, body shape, skin color, lip shape, or eye color. In addition, for exploiting an opportunity to get intimate, many men will show openness to various types of women. This is a consequence of the primary instinct and, some might even say, because of the genetic code that is in each of us. The opportunity of a new adventurous relationship could make many men ignore other aspects, such as the intellectual or cultural side of a woman. Still, such aspects could be quite relevant when it comes to a long-term relationship and personal fulfillment.

It is quite common that people who share similarities to attract each other. Thus, those who have the same education, hobbies, interests, and passions tend to frequent the same places and have better chances of attracting each other. If both persons appreciate the similarities between them, the body look and shape of the partner might play only a complementary role. In many cases, their similarities, common attitudes, interests, or hobbies could help a couple strengthen their bond far more than physical appearance.

People develop through different stages. This is why a man might manifest different needs and desires through his lifetime. In many cases, younger men will focus on fun, interesting, and adventurous relationships. Later on, many men seek personal fulfillment and stability. Commonly, marriage is the concern of men who have found love and fulfillment with a woman they love. During their lifetime, men have various aspirations and necessities. Their needs and desires differ also from man to man. There could be all kind of scenarios. It could be even young men searching for stability and marriage or older men searching for adventurous relationships.

For many men, their education is a key influencing factor on how they seek their partner and develop their relationship. Educational level could lead to different individual aspirations, perspectives, and needs. Many might consider education levels as milestones in the evolution of a person. Depending on his educational level, a man could aspire for a specific lifestyle. Even if most men will still be open to various partners, in many cases, the educational background could play a key role in his quest of finding his life partner. Therefore, it is quite common for a man who wants to develop a long relationship to consider more the educational similarities and background of a woman than her physical aspects. This does not mean that the physical aspect of a woman does not matter for him. It is just that many men are open and attracted by a wide variety of women's body types, and that the education level of a possible life partner could work in a woman's advantage.

The social status of a person also often plays an important role in building a relationship. When it comes to searching for a life partner, many men are under the influence of their social status. It is quite common for men to prefer women that have a similar social status and share similar interests. Even so, not all men are the same. There are men who do not care about the social status of their life partner and are more interested in the other traits of a woman, such as character or appearance.

Men have various preferences and desires. Some of them love what others do not. There are millions if not billions of unique preferences, dreams, and desires. You can be sure that there are many men, like us, who prefer curvaceous and plus-size women. So many men love and prefer curvaceous and plus-size women, in fact, that it would take more than a lifetime to count them.

How to attract and keep your man

Finding the one, perhaps the one-and-only one has always been a tricky thing in the mind of singles. No matter if you are young, inexperienced, or perhaps even a virgin or a mature person, woman or man, this is never an easy thing to solve. It might surprise some, but this has little to do with you having fat or curvaceous body. Actually, so many factors could affect your quest that it would be hard to combat the ones who summarize it as a matter of luck. I mentioned earlier a quest, because somehow I see this as one of the most important life quests of a woman or man—to find the one committed to stay with you for a very long time and know he or she will be there for you. Of course, when younger, there might be slightly different expectations, but those are not too different.

Now, how about curvy women and plus-size women? Many will say that is far easier for a skinner, slim-top, model-shaped woman to find and have her man, compared to a bigger or a plus-size woman. In some aspects, they could be right. Especially for teenagers, there are many cases when boys gravitate around the slim, skinny, and photo model-looking style of girls. Nevertheless, is their interest truly genuine? It could be, but I think rather not—I will detail that a little later. You should keep in mind that even if a woman benefits from a lot of attention and pretenders, it does not mean that is easy for her to find the one, just perhaps easier to find *any* one. This is quite a different thing. In addition, as you will learn later, there are other factors more important than having a slim and model-shaped body for getting the attention and interest of men. Many curvy and plus-size women already know this and benefit from a lot of attention from men.

As I was mentioning earlier, there is an important difference between finding your man, who will be the one for you, and having the attention and interest of men for whatever purpose. More or less, the same factors trigger success in both cases. No matter if you are searching for the one or just any one, you should be able to flirt and to conquer men.

Men, in many cases, are quite easy going about their sexual needs and quite receptive to flirting. Competiveness, ego, and sexual tensions contribute quite a lot to this. Still, notice that not all the men are the same. Even the same man will not always feel the same. It might be that a man who is quite open and eager to flirt today may not be in the mood at all the next day. In addition, because of their current relationships, many men could just not be interested at all in flirting.

Not all the curvy and plus-size women are the same. There could be women benefiting from their great body with great curves, which will help them in many cases to attract and decisively capture men's interest. On the other hand, what one man might consider uninteresting, another could find deeply attractive. In reality, there is a variety of scenarios and possibilities. This makes it quite hard to have a secret formula on how a woman could be successful. You could be too fat, or your shape to be less defined or too defined; you could be too tall or too short, to shy or too loud; you could like or dislike some things. Some men might find you appealing or not, showing you a lot of interest or none, depending on many other factors such as their taste, their availability, the specific situation where you meet them, what values and preconceptions they have, and so on.

There are many discouraging scenarios, no? Actually, some key ingredients could increase your attractiveness, sex appeal, and success in finding the one or keeping your man. Before getting deeper into this, let's talk about one of the most successful and powerful ingredients: your smile.

Attract men and flirting tips

Sometimes when a man smiles at you (in a genuine, polite, flattering, non-invasive, respectful manner) your mood and day could change totally. Did you care much that he was much taller or shorter? Was it important that he was a businessperson or sportsman, that he was younger or older? Perhaps these were not so important. Of course, he had to be a presentable and decent man, but sometimes not even this might matter. It all depends on the smile.

Well, with men is the same, with the slight exception that many men are encouraged to take action by your smile. Do not expect that all will take action, since many men are quite shy also. This depends on the culture and the place you are. In some places, men could be more reserved while in other places they could be quite invasive.

On the other hand, different men may interpret your smile differently. Nevertheless, this should not scary you in developing your own genuine smile. It does not have to be a killer smile like the one some actors have. Sometimes, a shy, almost invisible, simple, and authentic smile could be a thousand times more powerful.

What else could be relevant beside your smile? It is also about your gestures, facial expressions, and your eyes. Sometimes it is a matter of a simple movement of your hand through your hair, or it could be about how you position your eyebrows, lips, or legs. There are many books related to body language, which could help you to learn more about gesture and facial expressions and how to reveal your interest or availability to men. These books will also give you a glance at key feminine gestures showing availability and openness. Even if these books will not give you a secret formula to succeed; however, they may be an interesting and useful tool for you, helping you to be more aware of your appearance and to be slightly more in control while flirting with men.

A key factor while flirting with men is how you feel about your body. Most probably, if you have the feeling that your are extremely fat, or that your body shape is too unpleasant or too vulgar, or if you think that your body is far from perfect, your chances of success could be dramatically decreased. When you feel bad about yourself, your self-confidence goes down, and your attractiveness will go down with it. However, sometimes curvy women and plus-size women are attractive and appealing even when they are feeling bad about themselves, most probably because of the attractiveness of their bodies. Nevertheless, many men will be discouraged to flirt or to approach them in this case.

I do not say that women should not care about their body, or the way it looks and evolves. Just keep in mind that when you flirt or are interested to flirt with a man, it will not help you at all to stress yourself about your body. That kind of negative energy and loss of self-confidence will most probably work against you. The funniest thing is that in many cases, after an unsuccessful or disappointing flirting experience, some curvy and plus-sized women consider that the failure was because of their body, while actually it was because of their negative attitude and lack of self-confidence.

So, please, do not deny your body! Your body is the only one you have, and you cannot switch it. Most probably, millions of men on this earth would adore it if they had a chance. Of course, many curvy and plus-size women will try to get slimmer, or reshape their body. There is nothing wrong about this, as long you do it in a harmonious and common sense way toward yourself. Just remember that feeling bad or insecure about your body, together with a lack of confidence or enthusiasm, is totally a different thing than how your body looks. What is more important is that you control and positively influence your emotions and attitude, and this could have a tremendous impact on your life.

How about looking at him, and into his eyes? Would it be possible to flirt without making eye contact? It is quite hard to flirt without eye contact, as the eyes are one of the key factors in flirting. How do you know that he has a genuine interest in you without getting the confirmation from his eyes? By eye contact, you could confirm your availability and openness and you could encourage him to take action. Looking him in the eyes will also let you know if he is interested in you. Prolonged glances or eye contact will confirm both to you and to him your interest in each other. However, you should treat eye contact, especially prolonged glances, with caution. This is mainly because in some cases or cultures, men could interpret such gestures wrongly.

Coming back to flirting, how intense should your openness be? Will you need to have tons of enthusiasm, a large smile, and over self-confidence to be appealing? Well, actually you do not. Sometimes a shy, unclear smile and an even hesitant and slightly nervous gesture could be quite successful. However, these will most probably be even more successful if you are a positive, self-confident person, with a reasonable degree of self-awareness and control over your gestures. Also, keep in mind that in most cases, men need to be encouraged to take initiative and to talk to you. You will have to find the right balance between creating your desired appearance and ensuring he understands your signals, and that he is aware of your openness and availability.

Successful dating

How could you be more successful in dating? Well this is quite a hard topic for us, the authors, since when we think about it from our perspectives and experiences, in most of our first dates we were thinking about getting lucky. We did not always succeed at this, but many times the date itself was great, making us happy about it and self confident about ourselves. How about the curvy and plus-size women we dated in the past? Did they have to do something to be more or less successful? Thinking back, yes, there were some first dates where the women made the effort to increase their attractiveness. This does not mean that what they did could apply to all scenarios; however, the idea is worth exploring.

Many factors could influence your first date. These factors could be quite varied, such as what kind of man is he, what culture and values he has, what he does for living, how old he is, whether he is shy, what type of character he is, and so on. However, you should consider some simple things on your first date. Try to listen and understand him better, smile, and encourage his initiatives to the point where you feel comfortable and based on what type of relationship you will like to develop.

You should also try to find common hobbies and common things that you both like. Discussing topics you both enjoy will relax the atmosphere and could make your date a great one. Moreover, try not to overwhelm him with your problems. It might be a good idea to keep your problems to yourself and focus on the date instead.

A powerful strategy in the hands of many experienced women is playing hard to get. As with many other things in life, unavailable, limited, or hard to achieve things enhance desirability. However, before playing hard to get, you should be sure that it is appropriate and will not work against you.

Finding your love

How about love? Or love at first sight? Or making him truly love you?

First, do guys love curvy women, plus-size women, big girls or women? Definitely, yes! Many men love curvaceous and plus-size women. Why do many men love them? Love is not about the curves and the shapes of your hips. These might help you to be more attractive, but when speaking about love, it is hard to put your finger on specific physical factors. Men, or at least most of them, love women. That is how it has been for a long time, and that is how will be for a long time to come. The fact a woman is short or tall, thin or fat, younger or older should have little to do with love.

Love is the most important thing in a man's or woman's life. No matter if it comes quick or in time, we can hardly describe in words the greatness of love. Therefore, we will focus mostly on one key aspect.

How about if you fall in love and he does not like you, or he does not respond to you? Is it the end of the world? At that time, it might feel like it. It happens to many, many women and men in the world, no matter on their body shape. So what you can do about it? Sometimes you just might need to show him that you like him, but many times, he won't feel the same, and you will have to put up with it, no matter how hard you find it to bear. Believe us, if you are in this situation, it will pass.

Getting married

Do I want to get married? Will I get married? Does he want to get married? At what age should I get married? What kind of women do men want to marry? How do I get a guy to marry me?

These questions, at different times, might have enormous importance for many women. Is it easy to answer these questions? Not really. However, in many cases, the answer will have a lot to do with love, more exactly, returned love.

Love...and then marriage. It is quite hard to avoid marriage if there is love, especially for men. I am one of those who believed that as long as life partners are in love, those additional official papers and wedding celebrations don' t make sense. However, for many women, no matter how their body is, marriage is a key goal in life. Moreover, it is not just a simple goal for women; it also has a great signification, giving them the feeling of completeness. As a man, you have to find out, or be aware of, the importance and relevance marriage in your partner's mind. Then it is quite hard to ignore and not to take action. Even if I think that most men are not keen to get married, I might be wrong, since many male friends and acquaintances got married more from their own initiatives—at least they think so.

How about a curvy and plus-size woman? Is marriage much different in her case? Not really. As long there is love or a very strong connection, things should be similar. Now, could you do something to rush this as a woman? Definitely yes, since from my personal experience if it was not her actions I will postpone the marriage for eternity. There are men who are searching for this, and they will take the initiative. In this case, you will be a lucky woman—not like my life partner, who had to support my anti-marriage mood for many years. However, if you are not so lucky, and your friend is more or less like me, some of the tips below might help you, considering that there is a genuine relationship between you:

So what could you do to rush this moment? Below you can find some possible tips from my own experience; however, not all of them will be adequate for your situation or produce the desired effect. Therefore, it will be a good idea to reflect more on this and learn about your partner to ensure that your initiatives will be appropriate.

- Suggest to him (you should try without scarring him, as he might be sensitive about this) the importance and relevance of such a step for you.
- Ask him what he thinks about the idea of the two of you to getting married. Before

this, be sure that he knows or senses that marriage is something you desire.

- If after discussing this he seems to be OK with the idea, but sensitive or stressed about the event itself, try to make the event be, or at least to seem to be, a simple and quick thing to do and organize.

- Do not quit if there is no positive reaction from him. Come back to the topic after few months, or whatever period seems appropriate, without being pushy. Just ensure he knows the importance of this for you.

- If he has not discussed marriage, you should not be shy to open the topic for discussion. However, make sure that a relevant period has passed since you began your relationship, so that you will not scary or stress him from the beginning. Keep in mind that there are all kinds of men. In my case, it took my girlfriend ten years to bring me to this step.

- Be polite, sensible, and sensitive about marriage in your discussions.

If you are a curvaceous or plus-size woman, you should be aware that body shapes do not matter so much for being single or not. There are all kinds of single women. In addition, you should not despair because it is not the end of the world if you do not get married tomorrow. Even if you never marry, the world will not end. Look at how many celebrities are single or continuously divorcing. Rather than stressing yourself about not being married, you should focus more on feeling good about yourself, having fun and self-confidence, and taking care of your body and life while searching for the *one*. Sometimes, you might not need to be so demanding or perfectionist in this quest. A short look, or even a first date, will not reveal all the qualities of a man. Sometimes, it might take a lot of openness to find what you are searching for.

Keeping him

Some of the key ingredients for a successful long-lasting relationship are true understanding and genuine caring about the feelings and needs of your partner. Beside this, some salt and pepper—such as smiles, laughs, or from time to time arousing experiences—might bring some more color and life into your relationship.

Finally, in your quest to find the one, keep in mind that the world is large. There are billions of men and women, all kind of men and women. Some will like or search for something that others do not like. Therefore, you should not stick with one opinion or view. Open your mind and learn more about the world. There is an abundance of uncertainties, opportunities, dreams, desires, fears, and possibilities. You should try to look at love in a positive, self-confident way, and if possible, from time to time, with your unique genuine smile.

Food, diet, and body care

Do you need a perfect diet to lose belly fat or weight?

Do you really need to lose weight? Probably, most women will say yes. Nevertheless, do you really need to? Do you really need to spend so much of your energy, time, and thoughts on this? Should you keep searching for a perfect diet or strategy for becoming the desired weight? If you already have a diet in place, should you stick to it, or is there a better way?

The decision to lose weight or not should be entirely yours. However, keep in mind that apple, pear, and full-figured women's curves are quite sexy, and, not in only a few cases. Men see the body shapes of curvy women and plus-size women as gorgeous and highly appealing. So before investing much energy into a dietary plan, think about whether you really need to lose weight.

Losing belly fat or weight might be a good idea, sometimes even a must, if your current weight could bring health risks.

We have to recognize that many plus-size women enjoy an intense positive feeling after they have lost a significant amount of weight following a dietary plan. Their smile comes back and they feel more positive. There is a great effect on their minds and they feel much better about their body. They even feel healthier, charged with energy, and self-confident. Moreover, all of these feelings and attitudes highly contribute to their own self-perception, and more important, to the perception of others around them. However, do you really need to lose weight to feel good about yourself and transmit all that positive energy around you? That is for you to decide.

In many cases, if your body triggers a lot of inconveniences and you have health risks, losing weight might be an idea worth thinking. Still, there are many cases where many plus-size women have a healthy and beautiful body and they do not really need to lose weight. Even if, in these cases, losing weight might not be a bad thing, it might not be as important as many will think. Rather than investing all that energy into losing weight, it might be better to spend it on having a balanced and positive life with far more satisfactions. Moreover, the ironical part of this is that a balanced lifestyle also brings, in many cases, a balanced body weight, reducing the risk of becoming too overweight. It is like breaking the loop by focusing on the cause instead on the effect. By simply being aware that *you* are what is important and that your lifestyle and the way you feel about yourself matters the most.

No matter what, you do not have to wait to feel good and positive about yourself, especially if there is not such a critical need for losing weight. Do not postpone feeling good about yourself and try to smile every day.

The only woman I remember who had nothing to do with diet and losing weight is my grandma. I cannot remember or imagine her speaking about dieting or losing weight. Even so, this does not mean she did not have them on her mind or in her life. It is just that I cannot remember or imagine her stressing herself or spending lots of time and energy on her weight.

On the other hand, all the other women I know have dedicated some amount of time, energy, and importance to their weight. Indirectly, from time to time, even if I did not wanted to be, I was involved in their quest for losing weight and finding the perfect approach for it.

Weight loss and diet books

I learned about a lot of diets and approaches for losing weight from books, magazines, and women spending their energy on this topic. Sometimes, I had the feeling that women who desperately want to lose weight are entering into a sadistic never-ending loop without actually focusing on losing weight or finding a good approach for it.

Does it really matter to lose the weight? Most plus-size women might think that, in their case, it is very important to lose weight, especially when comparing themselves to slimmer women. However, all kind of women, with all kinds of bodies, stress themselves a lot over their weight, even if many of them have a very slim body.

Within this book, we will not try to recommend a perfect diet. Even if we feel tempted to discuss various diets, because of a good personal opinion or enthusiastic feedback we've received, we will not recommend a specific dietary plan. We will not do this because, as you might know, having a diet recommended to you will not solve your weight-losing quest so easily, especially if it is a lifetime quest.

Instead, we will try to focus on some key tips and ideas that will increase your chances of feeling good about yourself and losing weight in a smooth sustainable and harmonious way.

At present, many diets are suggested or recommended over the Internet, or in reference books. Some of the existing diets are more successful, and some might be more or less appropriate for you. There are also other choices, more or less appropriate for you, such as physical exercises or body- shaping wears.

However, before making your choice, keep in mind to choose a harmonious and healthy solution for your body. You should also consider getting advice from a professional in the field. In this case, be sure to check for references, credentials, and trustful reviews related to his proposed solutions.

The key success ingredients for most diets

We see losing weight as a matter of body care and health. In addition, we see it as a strange idea seeded deeply in the woman's mind, related to her attractiveness. No matter your reason, if you really have to lose weight, the ideas below might help you.

First, if you are feeling good about your body, you are healthy, and your weight does not increase health problems or risks, then perhaps you should not stress yourself about diets. Let other do this. However, you could still learn or pay attention to different diet plans, advice, and tips, but do not spend too much energy on them. Instead, spend more time on feeling good about yourself and having great quality moments in your life with yourself and with others.

How about the cases where you have gained weight in the last few years? This is quite a stressful scenario for many women; and many women in this case would like to go back to their previous weight, or, at least to most of the weight they gained. Our opinion here is that your decision to follow a diet plan and lose weight should come because of a real need to lose weight, not because your weight was lower in the past. You should consider if the weight is tough for your actual situation. Does it put you at risk for health problems? Does it really stop you from feeling good about yourself? How much time and energy do you have to dedicate to losing weight?

Before concluding, keep in mind that for diet success, the dietary plan should be comfortable for your body, good for your health, and OK for your mind. In addition, your diet plan should be one that, if necessary, you are willing to stick to your entire life.

During a diet, you should always be aware of balance. Let us suppose that you did chose a healthy perfect diet plan for losing weight, a plan that is perfect for your body type and health. If for any reason, you cannot stick with it—for example, one day you break it and eat many sweats—you should not get disappointed and treat yourself as a loser. Rather, treat this as an exception and focus on the long-term balance in your life since balance is far more important than some occasional disturbances. Keep in mind your overall goal, and, as long as it is good and healthy for you, stick to it, without being discouraged or disappointed by some exceptions along the way.

Attitude, humor, and self confidence

Attitude is the materialization of all thoughts, beliefs, and principles of an individual. Attitude, humor, and self-confidence have close links and interdependence. Attitude could be negative or positive. A positive attitude includes self-confidence, optimism, courage, and humor, while negative attitudes could include distrust, fear of failure, anxiety, or sadness. This outlines the idea that attitude contributes significantly to the overall image of any individual. Attitude is also important because we could differentiate people based on their attitude. Within our society, it is quite common to appreciate and prefer those who display a positive attitude. Optimistic and self-confident people naturally attract other people around them.

People generally influence each other. The attitude of the people surrounding us influences us. During our lives, the attitude of others, such as childhood playmates, parents, friends, life partners, and work colleagues could influence our own attitude.

The way we think, the principles we adopt, and our personal beliefs dramatically influence how we choose to act, behave, and react in society. Clearly, attitude is one of the distinctions between people, and in many cases, it is at the base of being a successful person or a winner.

In many cases, if not most of them, attitude is more important than appearance. For example, we may notice a person with a great physical appearance but who lacks a positive attitude. The natural reaction of many people is to avoid such a person, to keep a distance despite his/her attractive appearance. This happens because many prefer to be around people who have a positive attitude. It is not a surprise that happy and lively women with a good sense of humor and optimism attract many around them. Commonly, being in the company of such women is something pleasant and desirable, no matter of their physical aspects. In other words, it's not just the shape of her body that dictates the true beauty of a woman. Some might say that a positive attitude is an important part of feminine beauty.

Our attitude influences the perception of those around about us. It could be responsible for the reactions of sympathy and antipathy from the people around us. If you consider that nature was not quite generous with your physical traits, a positive attitude could be a real advantage and powerful substitute. Positive thoughts, optimism, and humor often create a good mood for the people surrounding us. Those who cherish a positive attitude improve the mood of others. Positive people could also inspire other people around them, hence people's interest in seeking those with a positive attitude. Many people prefer interacting with positive people and avoid the negative mindsets.

Apathy, anxiety, lamentation, and lack of self-esteem could be attributes of a woman with a negative attitude. When these characteristics are visible, surrounding people might react with avoidance or rejection. This happens because people are more open to positive persons who are able to maintain, enhance, or transfer good mood, inspiration, enthusiasm, or self-confidence.

Awareness of one's personal beliefs and principles could be useful to anyone who is unhappy about certain aspects of her life. We cannot expect a change in our lives if we think, act, and react in the same way every day. Instead, we could improve our way of thinking and our beliefs and attitudes. If we want a strong positive change in our lives, we might need to change our core concepts, beliefs, or the way we perceive reality. Changing our way of thinking, reassessing beliefs, and adopting new and healthier principles could lead to powerful results. When thinking about an attitude change, you should be aware and identify the seeds of optimism, courage, and self-esteem within you. In addition, you should try to avoid fear, lack of confidence, apathy, anxiety, and bad moods.

A positive attitude will cause a person to focus on identifying solutions for his issues or problems. Depending on your attitude, you could see the bright or the darker side of life. As an example, a negative attitude could be focusing on paying attention to the limitations and failures of others, rising problems, and criticizing. On the other side, a genuine positive person will look and search for positive aspects and opportunities even in darker scenarios.

A positive attitude could help you to attract good people around you. It could improve your relationships with colleagues and friends. In addition, it might play a key role during finding love and building a successful relationship. A state of contentment and satisfaction could enhance your self-confidence. Moreover, these are powerful drivers in attracting the admiration of others. In the presence of self-confidence, you could increase your joy of living and have far more successes. The experience of successes will strengthen your self-confidence even more. This might be a learning route toward a certain destination. Once you know the route, it might be just a matter of remembering the landmarks to know what to do in order to achieve the ultimate goal. Nurturing good humor, optimism, and self-confidence are key approaches for a positive person. In addition, by focusing more on our qualities and not on our defects, we create a stronger feeling of personal fulfillment. It is in the power of almost any woman or man to focus on the positive side of our being.

Positive results will appear in most cases when a woman focuses on her qualities. It is hard and sometimes impossible to admire a woman who does not have a good opinion of herself. As long as a woman will not feel good about her look or body, she will act accordingly, and most likely, others will not be able to perceive her any differently. By focusing their attention on their unique advantages or specific physical charms, most women could create a positive image and perception. The manner in which we look at ourselves plays a key role in how others see us. Therefore, as already mentioned before, what matters most is our own impression of ourselves. By focusing on our true qualities, most of us will positively influence our own perception of ourselves and others' perception of us. In conclusion, a positive attitude is one of the key ingredients that could lead us in the direction we want. Many might consider that attitude is at the base of our successes.

Do men prefer lonely women?

Spending more time alone could give you a good opportunity for meditation, self-reflection, and self-awareness. Many people appreciate and consider the intimacy of thinking important. This happens because of the need to focus on personal material or spiritual concerns. By taking time to asses and think about ourselves, we become more aware of our position in a social context. Therefore, to some degree, loneliness could be an opportunity to think and deeply reflect about our lives and about the people near us. By improving our knowledge and understanding about ourselves and about the people surrounding us, we understand easier how we fit in our society. By understanding others, we could improve the quality of our relationships with other people. When we see loneliness as an opportunity to understand others and ourselves, it could lead to good interpersonal communication.

Even so, there are occasions where loneliness is harmful and the intensity of self-concern works against us. If we show interest only for ourselves without relating also to the people around us, we might risk isolating ourselves. By not caring about the people around us, we risk unbalance or destruction of our social relations. In some extreme scenarios, others might start to marginalize us. It is in the nature of people to live together with others. Because we are social beings, we find it hard or even impossible to live alone. Therefore, in many cases, isolation of a person could have damaging effects.

Sharing ideas, values, principles, and beliefs with others can be very helpful for every individual. By communication with others, we can improve and refine our ideas and beliefs. It is quite natural for a discussion partner to add, contradict, or subscribe to your views. By communicating with the people around us, we improve our communication skills, self-confidence, knowledge, and horizons.

Many could see a social group as an assembly of people who share similarities, such as the approval of values, ideas, or beliefs. Sometimes, by belonging to a group, a woman could have an image as a flexible, thinking, and caring person. This could be because her connection to a social group might have, at the base, the acceptance of other opinions or ideas. In many other cases, the openness to listen and discuss the ideas and thoughts of others could provide an opportunity to develop a social relationship. You do not necessarily need to exclude your own principles or beliefs to belong to a group. Even so, if you intend to successfully be part of a group, it could be desirable to respect opposite ideas and beliefs.

By developing your communication skills within social groups, you increase your chances of better handling a personal relationship. For example, abilities like the flexibility to listen, the openness to understand other points of view, empathy, and caring could help you in your quest to find and keep your dream man. As a flexible and open-minded person, you could have a better chance to create a favorable environment and reach consensus with your life partner. The ability to show empathy could often help you avoid conflicts with your partner and find constructive approaches. By showing empathy and genuine understanding, you could increase your chances to find the man of your dreams or to have a long and healthy relationship.

By ignoring the ideas, principles, or beliefs of others you risk exclusion. We could avoid isolation by showing tolerance to others' ideas and opinions. Those who tend to think that only their opinions matter might not obtain the acceptance of others easily. It is quite common for such people to wake up alone. There are cases when loneliness has a more toxic and harmful effect and less benefits or stimulating effects. In specific cases, loneliness could even lead to conflicting or uncomfortable psychological states. Such a mind state will make it even more difficult to communicate or to have the acceptance of others. Many people try to avoid persons who show a rigid and negative attitude. In some extreme scenarios, this could even affect their status in society. Others might rather prefer to avoid such a person, instead of confronting her stubbornness or negative personality.

Even so, the skilful ability to communicate or to adapt to a group does not guarantee finding or maintain a personal relationship. There are communicative persons who can easily integrate into groups, but do not succeed to have a personal relationship. However, a communicative woman might have better chances to find and build a relationship. In addition, keep in mind that men are also less or more communicative. And men have various tastes and preferences. Some might prefer and like shy and introverted women, while others might feel the need for a more dynamic communication. There are many cases when the shyness of a woman triggers a powerful attraction from men.

Sometimes we have to be alone to realize and appreciate what it means to be together with someone.

Are you special enough?

All women are beautiful and special. Women prove to be stronger than men are in many situations. Women seem to be more aware of the surrounding reality. It is also quite common for a woman to show more concern for the welfare of the family. It might be because the maternal instinct or love for her children increases her willingness to compromise or to sacrifice.

A woman's life partner could make her feel even more special. In many situations, our life partners could influence how we perceive feel about ourselves. If we benefit from a clear appreciation of ourselves, we tend to behave accordingly. As a result, our self-esteem could grow and our actions might have more success. Such a feeling of personal satisfaction could be visible in our social activities. There are various ways to make the person near us feel great. Depending on the traits of our partners, their education, their character, and the nature of the relationship, there could be various ways to create a positive feeling. It might be admiration, appreciation, love, respect, or careful consideration of the lover, husband, family, colleagues, or friends. Any of these could cause most women to feel special enough. Each person that makes us feel special helps us to achieve a higher feeling of personal fulfillment.

People appreciate others for a reason. It will be hard for you to achieve appreciation of others by doing nothing. Many people admire others only when they offer something valuable in return. If a woman does not stand out in any way, it will be hard for her to get attention. Because of this, we might consider that each woman is responsible for the appreciation she gets from others. In other words by doing nothing, people will hardly find you special. The appreciation of a person at a given time could depend on her previous involvement, dedication, or efforts.

People might see you as special because of your way of being, your character, image, or way of thinking. Others might consider the way you communicate, listen, appreciate, or even love. It is quite common for people to show appreciation and openness to the ones who also appreciate them in return. Any woman could be special, regardless of how she looks. To be more special, you do not need to be the center of attention. These two aspects could hardly be similar. Seeking the spotlight often implies a superficial upbringing and material interests. Sometimes you could be in the spotlight because of a well-tailored dress, a trendy hairstyle, a good matching purse, or other smartly chosen accessories. But this does not equal a genuine feeling of appreciation from others. True appreciation seems to have deep roots in a less material area of our beings and requires a continuous attention and refinement over time. The way we live our lives and relate to others could make us less or more special.

The power could be found in your mind

The human mind could be both an ally and an enemy. Our attitude could influence the way we think. As long as a woman's attitude, regardless of her appearance, is positive, her mind will have a better chance to focus on and achieve success. In the case of a negative attitude, the mind might attract failure. Therefore, it is very important to pay more attention to the attitude that we adopt. The events in our life are often the result of our reflections. In addition, in many cases, we can see that positive thoughts contribute to a positive attitude. By adopting a constructive and positive way of thinking, a woman could have a better chance of reaching her goals. Positive thinking, together with the confidence in your own abilities, is, in many cases, indispensable in achieving success. Whenever we believe what we imagine is possible, we increase our chances to make it happen.

To increase her confidence a woman could focus her attention in those aspects that put her in a favorable light. In many cases, it is a good idea not to search for weaknesses and to ignore negative aspects. This might be useful because the nature of thoughts provides guidance for our attitude.

Regardless of the nature of our thoughts, our mind will be the one that contributes its realization. Sometimes could be in less favorable circumstances, without understanding how we got there. In such scenarios, it is quite common to blame someone or something. It is much easier to point with our finger outward than toward our selves.

Given the importance of our dominant thoughts, we might need to give more attention to these thoughts, to analyze them, and then to act accordingly. It is in the power of each of us to choose our way of thinking. We could chose to think more about things we like and less, or even ignore what we dislike or what makes us unhappy. In this way, we could create a good mood for ourselves. Such a good mood could lift the corners of the mouths of many women and make their faces shine. Thus, by having a friendly and pleasant appearance, one could have more chances to obtain the appreciation of those around her. When we smile at others, there is a big chance that they will smile back to us. It quite common if you offer a smile to get even more smiles in return. By initiating such a gesture in a generous way, without expecting something in return, you could achieve a genuine naturalness and far more appreciation from others. Such a principle could be applied in others aspects of life. For example, after we support someone without wanting something in return we could receive her or his help in far more complex or difficult situations. Behind such events could be the capacity to empathize and show good intentions. We might see such traits, in many scenarios, as key components of a positive attitude. As long as our focus remains on the positive side, there is a big chance that our actions and results will be positive as well. Thus, by focusing on a positive way of thinking and on the positive aspects of life, we reduce the relevance of the negative aspects from our lives.

In some realistic scenarios, the human mind may be able to make the impossible possible. Positive words might be able to feed your mind and to generate positive beliefs, while negative words could give birth to bad beliefs and cause failures. Positive beliefs provide a solid base for a firm attitude, confidence, and an optimistic approach to the challenges in our lives. Positive beliefs could make the dreams or ideas that appear in our minds have more chances to become reality. In other words, by treating the projects born in our minds with confidence and positivism, we are closer to personal fulfillment. In addition, we might be closer to know fulfillment's satisfaction if we are willing to believe strongly in goals and ideas. In addition, perseverance and sustained efforts help us see our ideas happening. We can hardly achieve our ideas, even the best ones, without confidence, perseverance, and efforts. Another key ingredient to our success is our commitment. We could see success in many cases as the result of our sustained actions, perseverance, self-dedication, and passion.

The only limits in our mind could be those self-imposed. Quite often, we see the world in terms of our limitations. Thus, in many cases, such a limitation could not be favorable to us. Some might say that the world will treat us as we watch it. The way we position in relation to others affects us; by having more constraints, we could have a less or more advantageous position in our society. It is quite probable that the results of our present are the effects of our way of thinking and acting in the past. Things like self-confidence, courage, initiative, and good humor could become habits and beliefs. Then they might move in the subconscious of a person, defining her character and naturalness.

In various situations, such a person could naturally react in a positive manner. By doing this, she could enhance her chances to achieve her dreams.

Sometimes we spend the same amount of energy, no matter the results. It is quite common for us to avoid, instead confronting our fears, challenges, or difficult situations. By overcoming our own comfort limits, we could have a feeling of uncertainty or even psychological distress. Therefore, many times, we abandon the idea of confrontation. In many cases, by not facing and avoiding life's obstacles, we give birth to and encourage negative beliefs. In this way, we diminish our own strength to move on and we tend to retreat into a dim corner of our consciousness. Even if some might consider this a comfortable and safe nest, it is far from a harmonious lifestyle. By isolating ourselves and not facing our challenges, we build the premises for distrust, fear of ridicule, sadness, helplessness, anxiety, or apathy. Living such a life, could make us miss favorable situations and think that everything is against us. Indeed, the brief moment after we avoid our challenges provides us some comfort and even good feelings. However, on the medium and long term, we might experience negative feelings, regrets, and even resignation. Missed chances and regrets could ultimately lead us in the unfriendly and hostile territory of resignation. At this stage, some of us become aware that we could create and exploit opportunities by facing the challenges from different stages of life. However, it is good to know that, sometimes, life pays ups as much as we demand and dare. You could imagine this, as in the example of two people negotiating. By aiming high and trying to achieve great goals, you will have better chances to achieve great results.

Sometimes, in order to achieve your goals, it will be necessary to identify those negative beliefs that sabotage you and to replace them with positive ones. In other words, we have to use our mind as an ally. First, we should be aware of the things that limit and constrain us, and then we will have to work to eliminate or replace them. Those who manage to make such changes commonly open their minds to novelty.

Such people might even succeed to replace reality with their dreams. Many of the people who innovated or opened new roads in our society were pragmatic dreamers. Many of their dreams become a reality that surrounds us today.

Not always, but often enough, by sticking to an idea or belief we will achieve success. Perhaps many of our ideas or beliefs have led us successfully through certain points of our lives. Even so, there is no guarantee that if we stick to them, they will do the same in the future. Therefore, a periodic review and evaluation of our ideas, viewpoints, and beliefs could make a difference. As long as our objectives change, our old ways of action might not fit the context anymore. To accomplish new goals and missions, you will have to consider new approaches. New ideals might require new plans and ways of action. Sometimes if you want to become what you wish, you might need to do what you have not done yet. By initiating such actions for achieving your goals, you will have to challenge your self-confidence, courage, ambition, and willingness. In many cases, this will only depend on you since hardly somebody else could be responsible for your happiness.

When we face new challenges, we might need to exit our comfort zone. Nevertheless, by successfully overcoming the obstacles of our lives, we will increase our courage, boldness, and self-confidence. This could bring us far more fulfillment and satisfaction. By confronting our problems, challenges, or obstacles, we increase our chances to reach success and fulfillment.

Do money and career matter?

We could see career as a substantial source of income, as a special status achievement within the hierarchy of a company, or as the results of a person's devotion in a specific work area. Career offers various levels of professional and personal satisfaction for many of us. And many see career as a main way for making more money.

A career could offer safety, financial independence, importance, self-esteem, and even power. Many people associate career in their minds with the idea of life success or fulfillment.

The career achievements could offer a feeling of equality and independence. Also, our careers offer the possibility to exercise our abilities and competencies and to obtain recognition for it. In work environments, both women and men could compete and show their expertise and skills, no matter if they are leadership, technical, sales, teaching, or presentations skills.

In the beginning of human society, we used money as a tool of trade. Before money, people used various exchange methods to provide the necessities of living. After its introduction, money easily found its place in society. Shortly after, various commercial activities emerged and all kind of roles appeared. Such an important role was merchants—people who knew how to make profit from buying and selling goods and services.

During that time, money forged itself into a key role in our society; it is almost impossible to replace it today with something else. Money earned its place, demonstrated its usefulness, and is present everywhere in our lives. We work in exchange for money, and we spend it for our daily living. Larger or smaller amounts of money will cover our needs of food, clothing, transportation, rent, energy, and many other things.

At present, there is a link between money and our lives. Within society, people do not have the same abilities and chances to make money. Some of us could earn large sums of money almost effortlessly, while others could struggle each day for much smaller amounts. Some might consider that this is because of our financial education and our perception about money. Often, the education or trainings of a person contributes to her financial achievements. Nevertheless, there are many success stories where the academic education was less relevant for financial achievements.

Financial education plays an important role in the formation of healthy concepts about money in general. We do not want to discredit the value of academic education or specialized knowledge. On the contrary, we support their importance in society. Anyhow, in many cases people do not learn in school about their personal money management. When dealing with their personal money, many try to imitate the handling models learned from their parents. Such a model could be less or more appropriate. Sometimes intuition jumps to rescue us in our decisions. Even so, we can actually absorb some useful financial management principles for better administration of our revenues from various sources. The balance between our incomes and expenses could be a consequence of such an education.

In the absence of financial education, perceptions about money could take many forms. Some might even believe that "money could be the root of all evil," while others might believe that "only money could bring happiness." Of course, people do not fall only in two camps—those who see the money with good eyes, and others who see it with bad eyes. The opinions about the meaning of money are very different from one person to another.

Money could also be a tool that offers options and alternatives to their owners. It is quite common for a person with more money, options, and alternatives to attract the admiration or envy of others. Many people are open and tempted to associate with those they perceive as powerful. Many see financial robustness as one of the best clues about the power of a person.

By achieving financial independence, a woman could be less or more attractive to men.

Depending also on their own financial situation, some men might find this appealing while others might be more cautious and unhappy. Sometimes the financial success of a partner could bring happiness in a relationship while in other cases it could create frustration and negatively affect the relationship.

Most probably, many men, if not most of them, would like the attention of powerful and rich women. But later, once a relationship is in place, contradictions might arise frequently. Inconsistencies in financial status, ideas, habits, and common interests could create obstacles and tension between partners. Even so, there are many happy couples, where the partners do not feel affected by their financial situation.

Self-confidence, the perception about money, or the conception of success could be the ingredients that boost a person into a successful position. Even if someone could hardly share such traits with others, that does not always matter; there are many relationships where partners have a different financial statuses. Some of these relationships are short, while others are long lasting and full of reciprocal satisfactions. One key reason behind the successful relationships of people with different financial positions is emotional involvement. Depending on the nature and intensity of the emotions and feelings, a relationship could have less or more difficulties because of the financial differences between partners. Also, educational level, common interests, and habits could reduce the relevance of financial differences. Emotions often prove to be stronger than reason or calculations. Even so, financial status differences could be a real barrier for many relationships in all kind of scenarios.

Some might see money as a ticket that they could convert into beautiful houses, expensive cars, jewels, and exotic trips. But a woman could also invest such a ticket in education, training, innovation, or helping others in need. How we use the money and for what purposes depends largely on us. Many consider that moderation is a virtue that is often lost when a person is responsible for the administration of large amounts of money. Other might agree that money gives power to their owners, and that they could use this power for good or not. Money influences the lives of most of us and shapes the image of many.

Many financially powerful people show concern for the people and communities in which they live and try to create a positive impact around them. In this way, there are using their financial position to initiate or support actions that prove their concern for others and society. Others might be less open about their image in society or about the welfare of others. Even so, many rich people need social recognition and care about the collective perception. By supporting various actions for their community's commonwealth, richer members improve their image and reputation among less wealthy community members.

For many people, considerable revenue could be the result of a successful career. Today many women and men devote much of their life to building their careers. Financial independence is an important goal for many, but there are also other benefits of career advancement. Other benefits could be work satisfactions, learning opportunities, or the recognition of one's work, results, skills, and competencies. In most cases, people get money for their work results, performance, efforts, passion, dedication, and involvement.

Along her career path, a person seeks more than money. In many cases, the appreciation, esteem, and respect of others could be even more important than financial rewards. Money is indeed important; it is responsible for ensuring a certain standard of living to which we aspire. Nevertheless, without consideration of others factors, the feeling of accomplishment could not fully exist.

Another important aspect is the time we dedicate to our jobs. There are cases when the time and energy spent at work over certain limits makes it virtually impossible to focus on other aspects of our personal lives. There are also cases where people do not show motivation at work and endanger their careers. Thus, it could happen for a woman to focus more on her professional life at the expense of the personal one. Each of us has a limited amount of time and energy. After we invest them in various actions, we will need time to recover them. Because we do not always have the same time, energy, and dedication for our professional and personal life, we have to decide how to spend these limited resources.

A person, who wants to achieve self-fulfillment and satisfactions in both their professional and personal life, might consider allocating the same time and energy in both directions. However, it is almost impossible to spend the same time and energy for both career and personal life. Also, the way we handle one aspect has a direct effect on the other one. By neglecting the personal life, a person could endanger the smooth running of his professional life. Therefore, many of us have the challenge to find the right balance between our professional and the personal life, without abandoning either of them. When we dedicate ourselves exclusively to our professional life, we will increase our chances for career advancement, work satisfaction, and rewards. However, this will reduce the time we spend with our life partner, friends, or family. In time, such an approach could seriously affect the quality our personal lives and in some scenarios even our health or career. Some might not find it easy to develop a successful career and to maintain the same amount of time in a healthy couple relationship. Even so, for reaching self-fulfillment, finding the right balance between career and personal life should be a key objective for each of us.

Friends, family, children, or lovers are some of the important achievements of every human in his/her life. Most of us subscribe to this statement. Therefore, the highest satisfaction of our souls has its origin in the quality of relationships with the people around us. However, all these relationships require time, commitment, attention, love, and dedication. Even if some people consider that they do not have the necessary resources, the ability to cultivate these relationships in an appropriate manner will result in achieving a fulfilled personal live. By reaching fulfillment and stability in our personal life, we could also fuel long-term success in our careers. Even so, many people will prefer to develop only their professional *or* personal life. Each of us should follow his/her dreams and goals in the best way we consider.

Many men and women admire or show interest for successful women and men. Most of us appreciate and aspire for the company and friendship of powerful and successful people. This could be because we admire their strength and personality or because of our own aspirations and dreams.

Who is plus size? What plus size means

Within this book, by "plus-size women", we are usually referring to women with plus-size clothing needs. Most probably, these women have a curvaceous body, with more fat, and bigger bodies.

There are many views and opinions about what numbers can be considered for plus-size clothes. Therefore, we leave it to you to decide if you consider yourself a woman with plus-size clothing needs or not.

Even a search on the Internet will reveal many views on plus-size clothing. Many accept these views and many do not. In many cases, the term plus size is about clothes for larger-sized people. Nevertheless, how large is this?

In some unofficial references or Web sites, plus-size clothing starts from size 14 (US) or 18 (UK); in others it starts from size 12 (US) or 16 (UK) or 14 (AU). Even the famous encyclopedia Wikipedia presents plus-size clothing as starting from various numbers in various scenarios, not having a clear common worldwide-accepted measurement at the date this book was written.

The term plus size in relation to clothing has been widely accepted and many clothing creators and shops use it. Some clothing markets have specialized brands and shops for plus-size women's clothing.

Because of various interpretations and the complex mixture of body characteristics, it is quite hard to affirm that a specific type of woman is a plus-sized woman. Therefore, we shouldn't always refer to the size guides for the best answer as to who is plus size. The best answer should be that the women herself decides if her clothing needs are plus size or not.

Also, the understanding of what plus size is differs in other scenarios. For example, a modeling agency could have a completely different understanding of the plus-size term. In their case, they might even consider plus size starting from sizes much lower than 14 (US) for female plus-size model requirements.

The world is large with lots of cultures and lifestyles. Therefore, things could differ significantly from one corner of the world to another. For example, there might be places where plus-size clothing starts lower and places where it begins higher. Cultural perceptions for many Asian communities, for example, might consider most American and European bodies quite large.

How to be more attractive to men: Plus-size clothing ideas and tips

For lots of women, no matter if they are plus size or not, finding the perfect fit is sometimes a never-ending lifetime quest. Moreover, everything tends to be slightly tenser in the case of plus-size women.

How about appropriate clothes? Who should define what is right, appropriate, or good for you to wear? Should you use tips and suggestions you find in books, magazines, and over Internet? How about fashion trends that some designers introduced for plus-size women? Should you follow the tone and dressing style set by other plus-size women around you? Should you just follow your intuition?

Are any of the approaches above more successfully, especially when trying to attract men? Well, the answer is that it depends. In some cases, any of these approaches could give you a boost, improving your look. However, you should consider also that besides finding a good clothing style, there is something else as important as your clothes. That is how you feel about yourself and your attitude. With the right attitude and confidence, some women could turn a less appropriate clothing outfit into glamour. In the same way, with a serious lack of confidence and an inappropriate attitude, your outfit might make you shine.

Clothing has always been important. No matter what some might say, taking care of your look will increase your chances in many cases. However, keep in mind that, even if appropriate, clothing is an important part of who you are. There also are other things that contribute to your image or success; these are body care, attitude, self-confidence, the context where you are, and pure chance.

There are opinions, tips, articles, and advice in various media about how plus-size women could dress more successfully. We were not too surprised to find some common ideas repeated in the discussions we had with many plus-size women, especially related to the shape of the body:

- Apple-shaped body – a rounded body with the weight concentrated in the middle of the body. As an example, a great idea for many apple bodies is wide trousers or high-waistline skirt.

- Pear-shaped body – a body shape that slightly resembles the shape of a pear, with the bottom bigger than the top, in many cases with narrow shoulders. One great dressing idea for pear-shaped bodies could be an a-line skirt with a lower waistline. Wide trousers, especially in boot-cut and flare-leg styles, could be also a great choice for many pear-shaped bodies.
- Full-figured / shaped body – A good casual outfit choice for many fully figured bodies is a cotton or silk sundress. Another possible great idea is a pair of cotton capri pants and a denim jacket.

Before getting deeper into the clothing topic by revealing all kinds of clothing ideas that might be appropriate for you, keep in mind that all women are beautiful and clothing should suit your needs. By suiting your need, I mean to keep in mind that you are more important than the clothes itself. You will have to find a comfortable clothing style that you like and that fits you well. It is not as if the clothes are searching for the right sized woman, you are searching for the right clothes for you. If they do not fit your body and if they cannot be tailored to fit, skip them and find the right ones for you. No matter how much you like the model or how cheap it is, you should chose wardrobe clothes that fit comfortably to your body. Instead of forcing your body to fit into a smaller size, spend more time finding a comfortable outfit.

Do materials, colors, and patterns matter?

When it comes to colors, there are some general ideas for curvier women. Most larger women wear black or a darker, simpler color on the bottom or on the bigger part of the body, especially in the case of pear-shaped bodies. There is also the idea of using vertical stripes on the bottom and avoiding horizontal ones.

Are these ideas accurate? Do they really help you, especially when thinking about men?

Well, it could in some cases. However, you should keep in mind that many men love your body curves and shape a lot. So trying to hide your curves might not be always a good idea. Personally, I have seen very attractive plus-size women wearing white skirts or trousers. I also found a great outfit to be trousers made from a thin material, such as cotton, which are not narrow on the lower part of the leg. During summertime, many men like patterned, colorful, or light-colored sundresses on fully figured women. Many men like the shapes and curves of plus-size women. Of course, you will have to keep a balance between your voluptuousness and overall appearance. Sometimes showing too much in some areas might work against you, making you slightly vulgar.

When speaking about materials or fabrics, there is not a perfect one. It depends on lots of situations. Where do you intend to wear the clothes and show your beauty? Is it at the office? Is it a less formal environment or a party? If you are thinking about an informal outfit, a skirt or dress denim might be a good choice. In many scenarios, cotton will also be a good choice. For skirts and dresses, you could consider light materials such as silk. For some outfits, such as swimsuits or shirts, it might be a good idea to invest in better fabrics. By choosing higher quality materials, you will avoid early clothes depreciation, and your clothes will keep their smooth look on your body for a longer period. It might be quite inconvenient and unpleasant for your outfit to look baggy or worn after a short time, especially if we consider swimsuits or special occasion outfits. In the case of lingerie, silk might be a great option.

There are many great possible material ideas such as short or long denim skirts, velvet skirts, denim jackets, chiffon beaded dresses, and so on. For winter, a cotton top together with a cashmere coat and a pair of wide leg denim jeans could be an adequate choice. Depending on the situation, many materials could work for you. Therefore, you should consider trying all kind of outfits before actually making your choice.

Also, remember that no matter what color or material is your outfit, your attitude and self-confidence matters a lot. Your attitude and self-confidence could make your outfit shine or not.

Plus size stylish, trendy, and designer outfits

How about the plus-size clothing market? Are there many options for you? Leaving aside that the numbers on the labels might mean different things for different designers, not all the clothing designers have jumped onto the plus-size clothing bandwagon. There are many who still focus their new clothing collections on very small sizes, not giving you many buying options from their collections. That is mainly because the mainstream media is pushing so hard to associate beauty with slim and thin women. Moreover, many designers, who benefit and are dependent on media exposure, no matter how courageous they are with their collections, might not feel comfortable creating plus-size fashion. This should be their problem, not yours. They are constrained by media prejudices and have a narrow view. From our point of view, plus-size women are, in many cases, beauty itself. In addition, there is a big chance for these designers to lose a lot by sticking to their current views of beauty and fashion. However, many have turned around and started to recognize the beauty, value, and potential of plus-size women. This change might be, in many cases, because of money potential in the market, but nonetheless, plus-size beauty will be widely appreciated.

Where should you search for trendy and stylish plus-size designer clothes? The easiest way should be on the Internet. On the Internet already are many plus-size clothing catalogs. Many of these catalogs are also available offline. Before deciding on a specific catalog or designer, be sure you have considered others as well and that you did not choose the first one you saw.

In conclusion, you should love your curves and body shape, because most probably, many men will adore them if they had a chance. You should also pay attention to clothing styles and fashion trends, allocating your time to search for existing plus-size designers' collections to find your own personal clothing style; and once you found it, enjoy it and do not be shy to tell the world about it.

Plus-size dresses and skirts

First, it is quite clear to me that many plus-size women avoid dresses and skirts, especially shorter skirts. Many women tell themselves that after they lose a specific weight they will try it. Well, this is very strange to us and even if we understand how women make this decision, we do not agree with it in most cases. That is because the sexiest, most attractive women we have seen in dresses or skirts were plus-size women. We have seen curvaceous big women looking great in both short and long skirts. Even so, before deciding on short or long skirts for your wardrobe, you should spend more time trying various models and realistically choosing the ones that give you the most advantage. You should put aside any preconception that you might have. You should feel proud of your body and just try many models to figure out which longer or shorter skirts could bring you more advantage. While trying various skirt models, keep in mind that the most important thing should be how you feel about how you look. Try to spend less time considering what others might think about your look. Of course, you will have to keep a balance between satisfying your desires and considering how others might see you in an outfit. Nevertheless, the most important factor should be your opinion and feelings.

It is hard to shift a mindset. There are a lot of mainstream media and cultural influences out there, which make it difficult to convince many of you that plus-size women could look gorgeous in a skirt or dress. Of course, as in any other woman's case, you will have to find the right ones for you and the appropriate fitting for it. However, this outfit might not be so challenging and hard to find, as many women might tend to think. First, you should relax, trust in yourself, and try it. While considering various skirts or dresses, keep in mind where you intend to wear them. Also, for example, an A-line dress might be a very good option for apple or pear-shaped bodies, while a pencil dress might look great on some busty women.

Sometimes a simple classical or vintage dress or skirt might look wonderful on a plus-size woman. Even if some women might not prefer such an outfit, such a skirt or dress outfit could do wonders. That is because in some cases, the shapes and curves add value to it, giving it a smooth feminine and sensual look.

We do not agree the idea on focusing only on darker skirts or dresses to make your body look slimmer or balance the proportions of your body. We have seen many curvaceous plus-size women, more or less fat, big women, or fat girls dressed with light or colorful dresses or skirts, and they looked great. Keep in mind that light-colored or colorful dresses might be a great choice for your wardrobe, and you should not feel intimidated by your dress size needs. There are many great choices for all kind of dress sizes including 2x, 3x, 4x, 5x, big sizes, or maxi dresses, and so on. Just drop aside your preconception and spend some time searching and trying various models.

Below you can find a list with plus-size dresses or skirts ideas we tend to like. Some of these ideas might work for you; some might not be quite adequate for your case. These are only a few suggestions. You should also do a search by yourself to find more possibilities, and finally the right and perfect outfits for your body type.

Possible ideas:

- V-neckline, long floral dresses with back zip
- Solid-colored knit dresses with adjustable or twisted shoulder strap
- Maxi dresses in gradient colors, starting from a lighter color to a darker color at the bottom
- Knit dresses with short sleeves and small details around the neckline
- Purple, gray, or dark red tank-belted dresses with layered skirts
- White embroidered v-neck dress with knee-length skirts
- Floral or dark, short-sleeve, square-neck, knee-length dresses
- Navy, dark gray, or light blue v-neckline, layered denim dresses with elastic waist
- V-neck long sun-dress
- Knee-length, light- or dark-colored peasant formal dresses

- Colorful summer sun dresses with friendly bra straps
- Spring or summer strapless dress with light mixed colors and a flowing skirt
- A-line, v-neckline, floral dresses with a high-waist skirt
- Navy, dark gray, or light blue plus-size denim miniskirts
- Pin-up style cotton sun-dresses
- Dark red, dark green, pink, purple, or black strapless gown (prom dress)
- Black strapless designer gown/ dress for special occasions such as cocktail, party, club, or prom
- Beaded trim, black night dress for special occasions, floating around waistline
- Navy, dark gray, or light blue long, denim skirts might be a perfect choice for a winter casual outfit
- Olive, dark red, purple, gray, black, orange or navy plus-size sweater dresses as a great choice for autumn fall or winter wardrobe

- Beaded or embroidered skirts and dresses could be a perfect choice for many plus-size women looking for a special occasion dress
- Dark red, dark blue, or sapphire velvet dresses might make quite an impression on special occasions
- Plaid brown or dark-colored skirts with side zip
- Light-colored sleeveless skirt-dresses with a-line tulle skirt and adjustable straps
- Black or dark brown pencil skirt, ending slightly above the knees, with assorting belt
- Patterned or floral, black and white halter dresses
- Long, denim shirt dresses with details
- Fully-lined, dark-colored dresses with scoop-neck and long sleeves
- Dark red v-neck, long, beaded maxi dresses with shirring
- Brown, ruched, medium-sleeve, dress, ending below knees

- Floral gray, brown, pink, purple maxi dresses with lace-up trim
- High contrast-colored print dresses with pleated shoulders and long sleeves, ending above knees
- Light-colored print, maxi dresses with adjustable straps and shirring

So feel free to try many approaches until you find your own personal style. Keep in mind that you should chose a style that is comfortable for your body and you should have confidence for showing it to the world.

Plus-size pants, jeans, and shorts

As mentioned in the previous chapters, it is not such a good idea to force your body into smaller size clothes. It is not worth and it does not pay out. Instead, do some more searching, try more options, or even consider having your clothes tailored for you.

Wide-leg or boot-cut trousers and jeans, falling with a straight line on the leg might be quite an adequate choice, sometimes even the best choice for pear or apple-shaped plus-size women. Why should you not wear narrow trousers? In many cases, trousers that are narrow on your legs will show your body shape even more. Even so, narrow trousers might not always be a bad choice. Low-rise, skinny-fit jeans are also a great choice in many cases. You should focus on balancing your look while keeping in mind your overall appearance. Wide trousers can still show off your curves and body shape, and choosing them instead of narrow trousers might accentuate your voluptuousness too much in some cases. However, it is up to you to figure out which is the best option for you and which works more for your appearance.

While thinking about summertime or beach wardrobe, you might consider various models and colors of board shorts. Together with tankini, bikini, or a tank top, it could create a smooth appearance on the beach.

Plus-size tops, shirts, sweaters, and blouses

A general idea for apple-shaped plus-size women is to wear tops with a neck in v-shaped line. The v-line has the potential to highlight positively the upper part of the body, especially for apple-shaped and bustier plus-size women.

While choosing your top, be honest with yourself about your sizing needs. Then chose the appropriate sizes, no matter what the mainstream media might try to convince you.

Another strategy for bustier women who want to minimize focus on the top area could be to reduce the appearance of the top area through use of clothing and color in the lower parts of the body.

Sometimes long shirts and blouses could evidence the waistline of many pear-shaped plus-size women, but in some specific cases, even smaller tops could work well.

Pay attention that your tops and shirts are not very tight in certain areas. They will have to fit nicely in key areas of your body. Try to avoid giving the impression of "popping out."

Some possible ideas to consider, which could be less or more appropriate for your body type include:

- White or light-colored baby doll tank tops with shirring along the neckline
- Dark red, brown, navy, purple, pink, black, or gray cotton, v-neck, sleeveless tank tops
- Kimono tunic tops with sleeves
- Cotton tunic tops with long sleeves
- Beaded tunic tanks
- Satin trim, sleeveless tanks

- Long-sleeve belted cardigans
- Three-quarter sleeves, cowl neckline tunics
- Long sleeves, layered v-neck sweaters
- Long sleeves, cotton-embroidered sweaters with scoop neckline
- Long-sleeve cardigans with pockets at hips and open front
- Cashmere long-sleeve v-neck or crew-neck sweaters
- Long-length, medium-sleeve shirts
- Long- or short-sleeve plaid shirts
- Ruffled, stretch, short-sleeve, buttoned shirts
- Long-sleeve, buttoned shirts with straight pointed collar and countered shoulders
- White, light pink, or light-colored point collar, buttoned, cotton shirts with three-quarter sleeves
- Floral, buttoned shirts with straight collar and short sleeves
- Light blue, sleeveless ruffle shirt

Plus-size suits and costumes

Dressing for the office has always been a drag for women, especially for plus-size women, who in many cases have far more limited options. You should keep in mind that if some well-known designers or clothing shops do not have the right clothes for you, that does not mean you should feel bad about your body. There still are many ways for you to find yourself a perfect fitting suit or costume. Also, try not to force it. Do not try to fit yourself into a smaller suit or costume just because you think there are no options for you or that you will look slimmer. You should not force your body to wear smaller sizes, since it could seriously affect both your mind and health. Instead, you should spend more time finding a comfortable and perfect solution for you.

If you feel like there is no option for you, and you are close to the point of being desperate, just take a break, breath, and think again about a solution. A simple search over Internet could reveal many possibilities related to models, colors, patterns, materials, and so on. Relax and then try to find the right approach to finding the perfect suit, or even to having it created for you. It does not have to be from a very well known designer or shop; it just has to fit you as good as possible, feel comfortable, and be something you like.

Forcing yourself to dress in smaller sizes because you like a particular designer who does not create bigger sizes is not an option. If you struggle yourself, perhaps you will succeed to dress in such a suit or costume. Even if you succeed, you should consider with what it costs you to do it. If your clothes are too small for your body, you will feel squashed by them, and your body will not feel good or comfortable. In some cases, this could even lead to serious health problems, bad moods, or unhappy feelings. Dressing comfortably while at the office is important. If your clothes press in on your body and you feel uncomfortable, it will be quite hard for you to enjoy the good moments during the working day or focus on your career path. So even if it is quite tempting and seems convenient for you to try to squeeze your body into a smaller suit size, do not do it. Instead, spend some more time and energy finding a suit that fits your body well and that you like. Moreover, this will pay off, as you will feel much better during the time spend at work and on your way to the job. It will bring you far more satisfaction and self-confidence. Some plus-size women might think that if they succeed in squeezing their body to fit into a smaller suit, they will look slimmer and automatically sexier or more appealing for men. This is not necessarily true. From our experience, dressing in a much smaller size will not make a plus-size woman looking much slimmer or sexier. Dressing in inappropriate sizes could make your body look strange, and might show some key areas of your body in an unpleasant way. Some parts of your body might look like they are going to pop out. This, together with the fact that most probably you will feel uncomfortable, will trigger a lack of self-confidence. All of these could seriously affect your attractiveness. So believe us that it is not worth it to stress your body in this way. Instead, try to find a way, even if it will take you more time, to locate a comfortable suit or costume. There should be many options around you, just try to search the

Internet for plus-size suits. Also, keep in mind that you always have the option to go to a tailor to help you with this.

How about skirts? Do you have to wear only trousers? Even if a wide pair a trousers, falling down in a straight line, might look great on you, you should also consider a skirt. While considering a skirt for your office suit, a good option could be a skirt that ends slightly below, and in some cases above, your knee.

For bustier plus-size women or fully-shaped bodies, you should pay attention that the shirt fits properly and that it is not too tight in some areas. The shirt should nicely fit your body, and there should not be areas where the buttons look like they are going to pop.

We always feel surprised that women consider high heels necessary to be attractive. In some work and office environments, it might be less appropriate to wear very high heels. Moreover, it might surprise you that many men find flat shoes or shoes with lower heels quite attractive. You should not have a pre-defined idea that flat shoes are not modern or appealing; there are many interesting and great flat shoes. I have always considered classical and simpler flat shoe designs pleasant, despite many women who might think they are not pleasant enough.

While dressing for the office, you should also consider the formal or less formal dress code. Even if there is no policy on dressing, you should pay attention to how your colleagues are dressing and you should try to fit in harmoniously. This does not mean you cannot try more modern or courageous suits or fashion trends. Just be sure that your look does not contrast too much with the ones of your colleagues, or makes them uncomfortable.

A common office issue for some plus-size women is that sometimes they look too voluptuous, too sexy, or too hot. This could happen because of their pronounced curves or ample bust area. Is this good or bad? Well, in some cases this might work for you, and in other cases, it might work against you. Your appearance should depend on the scenario itself. What colleagues are there? How do they usually dress? How is the work environment? Are there dressing guidelines or policies? Are you intentionally showing too much of some key parts of your body? Is it too vulgar?

In addition, do not forget to try clothes on before buying. This will improve your chances of finding the perfect clothes for your body.

Plus-size evening wear for women

How hard is to find plus-size designer eveningwear, such as gowns or dresses for your body type? Perhaps many plus-size women will consider that their case is quite a special, unfortunate situation, not allowing them many choices.

If you think that your options are limited, you are wrong. Many beautiful outfits could make you stand out. Just drop the preconceptions you have and let all your choices be revealed to you by a simple search over the Internet. Even if your preferred designer does not give great options for your body type, there are many possibilities to dress your curvaceous body with a great evening outfit. No matter if you are searching for plus-size evening dresses or for formal evening gowns, there should be many elegant, classy, and even slimming evening dresses options available over the Internet. Some of these options might be less or more appropriate for your body type. However, following some more research, you could find your evening outfit.

Plus-size special occasion wear – cocktail, party, nightclub dresses, and tops

Below, you can find a list with special occasion clothes ideas. Depending on your body type, some of them could be great choices:

- Empire waist, a-line, v-neck, beaded straps, floor-length, special occasion dresses; great color choices: dark red, plum, navy, white, black
- Satin dresses with v-neck, v-back, flutter short sleeves, empire waist, a-line skirt
- White, light-colored, pink, purple, dark red, orange, or blue floor-length dresses, flowing from empire waist, with mid-back and halter neckline and beaded embellishment
- Fully-lined, floor-length gowns, with a dropped waist, strapless neckline, and mid-back, and beaded skirts
- Special chiffon dresses with v-neckline, pleated bodice, friendly bra straps, mid-back, empire waist, and ruffled skirt, ending slightly below the knee

- Silk knee-length dresses with v-neck, v-back, a-line skirt with empire waist
- Satin natural waist, high-back dresses with v-neck and a-line skirt, ending slightly above the knee
- Floral a-line dress, with short sleeves, empire waist, and knee-length skirt
- Long dresses with fully-embroidered skirt, bra-friendly knit bodice, v-neckline, v-back
- White, brown, dark red, blue, or light-colored a-line dresses with simple chiffon halter neckline, mid-back and skirt, ending slightly above the knee

Plus-size gowns, robes, chemises, and camisoles

Do gowns or robes influence how attractive men are finding you? Depending on the scenario, they could affect your attractiveness. Below are some possible ideas to consider for your wardrobe. Some of them might be less or more appropriate for your body and style:

- Sheer chiffon, semi-transparent, short-length, black or dark red robes
- Black or dark red kimono-style sleep-wear satin robes used together with a baby doll chemise
- A combination of a satin robe with adjustable straps and chemise
- Black, red, or navy satin nightgown robes with chemise lace trim and adjustable shoulder straps
- Darker-colored lace, long nightgowns, with high-cut leg, sheer lace, embroidered, and semitransparent details
- Purple, brown, navy, or dark red satin chemise with adjustable straps

- Dark, sapphire, or jade-colored lace trim nightgowns with adjustable straps
- Dark-colored cotton nightgowns with v-neckline, empire waist, and adjustable back straps
- Satin, floor-length lace gowns with lace trimmed cups, low back, and thin shoulder straps in a cross on the back
- Floral, embroidered chemises with contoured adjustable cups and ruffle at bottom
- Satin, floor-length gowns with low neckline tied with thin straps at the back and high-detail embroidery on the front and in the bust area
- Scoop neckline, v-neck camisoles
- White or light-colored semitransparent chiffon nightgowns with beaded lace trims, v-neckline, ending slightly below the knee
- Purple, satin, lace-top gown, beaded, with adjustable straps

Plus-size swimwear, swimsuits, and bathing suits

Before getting deeper into this topic, we have a small suggestion for large breasted plus-size women. It might not be quite clever to wear a smaller size bra. Your breast could look far more smooth and attractive if you avoid fitting your breast in small sizes.

Even if we've said this before, keep in mind to be proud of your body and feel confident about yourself. Many men out there prefer plus-size women. Also, while going to a beach or pool, keep in mind that you are OK, and that your body shape and curves could be attractive and pleasant for lots of men.

Regarding a swimming outfit, in many cases, for busty or fully-shaped, plus-size women, a one-piece swimming suit could be a very good choice. Be sure you have tried it before buying it, in this way ensuring that it fits properly, comfortably, and is smooth on your body. Feeling comfortable in the swimming suit should be an important factor when you decide to buy it.

As in the case of other clothes, there is the idea that black or darker colors will give you a slimmer look. We do not agree with this idea. In addition, you should feel good and confident about yourself, daring to wear more colorful and exotic colors. With self-confidence and a positive mindset, this will make you feel much better about yourself.

Is it easy to find a well-known designer bikini swimsuit available for plus-size bodies? Not really, since not all fashion designers have their creations available for all sizes. Nevertheless, there should be many sleek models and available options. You will just have to spend some more time looking until you find the perfect choices for your body type. Keep in mind that during your search, it is not always a good idea to search in stores for plus-size swimwear on sale. Sometimes there are some unpleasant reasons why those swimsuits are so cheap. In addition, you should pay attention that the materials are of quality. Avoid buying swimsuits mad of cheap fabrics that will lose their sleek look and sometimes even their colors after wearing them few times. Pay attention to the details related to quality and fabric before making your decision. If possible, it will help you to try them before buying.

Another option for plus-size women could be the tankini or blouson-style suit. This could be a good choice in the case of many plus-size women, especially for apple or pear-shaped bodies. You will have to try it and figure out if it is for you.

In many cases, a swimwear top or cover up could be an elegant, convenient, and beautiful choice. There are many attractive, flattering, stylish, and comfortable available options, such as:

- Floral blouson tankini tops
- Darker-colored, v-neckline halter tankini tops with adjustable tie
- Empire waist swim-dresses with double tank straps

- Strong-colored, v-neckline, short-sleeve, braided belt swim cover-ups
- Light-colored semitransparent beach tunics, ending slightly above knees, with long sleeves

Plus-size women with larger breast might consider a swimming suit with a built in bra.

Plus-size coats and jackets

Some of you might consider a coat or jacket not having too much to do with how appealing you could be for men. Indeed, when charged with lots of positive energy and a charming attitude, some personalities will be able to shine despite a less fitting outfit. Nevertheless, while choosing your wardrobe, you should dedicate time to choosing the right coats and jackets for your body type. This will increase your overall appearance and attractiveness. In addition, in many cases, it will have a direct effect on your attitude and state of spirit.

Among many available options for plus-size women's outfits, you could consider some of the choices below. A simple search over the Internet will reveal many blogs and sites presenting many more ideas to consider:

- Buttoned, dark-colored, rolled-sleeve blazers
- Sleeved jacket with ruffle front and zip closure
- Lightweight swing jackets for formal activities or work
- Buttoned, colorful cotton stretch blazers
- Long-length, buttoned denim tunic jackets
- Lined and pocketed leather jackets, with long sleeves and zip closure
- Patterned, belted, cotton, plaid jackets, with front pockets
- Lightweight, buttoned trench coats, with long sleeves, notch collar, and adjustable tie belt
- Strong colored, classic wool pea coat
- Plaid, knee-length trench coat
- Long, wool, fully-lined coats could be stylish winter outwear

- Dark-colored, buttoned, cotton fleece-lined jackets
- Colorful or patterned cotton-lined swing coats with three-quarter-length sleeves could be a great choice for spring or autumn

Plus-size wedding and bridesmaid clothes

We tried hard to find and to agree on some ideas for this key event in every woman's life. In this case, you should stick to your desires and dreams, but at the same time be realistic about your size. Search, try various models, feel comfortable about yourself, find what you like, know yourself, and be realistic about your measurements. Finally, have it tailored to make it as you imagine it to be.

Do not be frustrated if a dress you like does not fit. At least you have an idea of what you want for this special and unique day, and with some effort and further search, you will find a solution to have your dream dress for your special wedding day.

How about the bridesmaid? What could be a great plus-size bridesmaid outfit? Depending on your body type, there are many possible available ideas such as:

- Satin lace, strapless, fully-lined dresses, ending slightly above the knee
- Stretch dresses with lined bust and unlined skirt
- Beaded mesh satin halter dresses
- Stretch, knee-length, waist-banded dresses with lined bust
- Stretch halter dresses with ruche ruffle
- Lace, fully-lined halter
- Formal satin and chiffon gown with adjustable shoulder straps
- Colorful stretch satin, long dress with ruche
- Stretch, dark dress, with pleated skirts and spaghetti straps

Plus-size shoes and boots

Even if there are so many plus-size shoes and boots options available over Internet, we recommend searching in offline stores. Before buying a pair of shoes or boots, you should also try them. We do not recommend being satisfied with a simple and quick tryout of one shoe. Instead, ensure that you've tried both of them with the socks or stocking normally used in your future outfits.

Even if some models will be quite emotionally attractive for you, be sure that they are comfortable for your feet before buying them.

Also, keep in mind that sometimes a simpler shoe could contribute even more to your outfit, creating a pleasant and beautiful appearance. Sometimes flat shoes or boots could make your outfit far more attractive and appealing compared to huge heels by well-known designers, with details all over it.

How about plus-size lingerie?

Well, this is a topic were we feel more connected as men. Why? It might be because lingerie has always attracted attention and driven the imagination of many men. Besides giving you comfortable feminine feelings, lingerie has the potential in many scenarios to accelerate and arouse your partners' desires even further.

Is it easy for a plus-size woman to strengthen her look by choosing specific lingerie? Well, this depends on what type of lingerie you are speaking about, how it fits your body, your partner's tastes, the occasion you are using it, the fitting style you choose, the fabrics or materials, and so on. Nevertheless, in many cases, lingerie has the potential to bring your partner literary to your feet.

While you choose your lingerie, you should be realistically aware of your sizing needs and on what key body areas you want to show off. If possible, try before buying an item or at least before buying more items.

You should avoid lingerie items that are not your size. Getting the appropriate and comfortable size is quite important. For example, if you think about buying bras or hosiery, make sure they feel comfortable, that they do not squeeze you, and that they do not fall or roll down easily. Even if a corset could be a good idea, you should not choose one if it is not comfortable for your body. Squeezing and forcing your body to fit should not be your choice.

There are many alternatives and options for plus-size lingerie, both in shops or online. With a simple search over the Internet, such as "plus-size lingerie," you could access lots of plus-size lingerie in online stores. There you will have access to many lingerie items and clothes, such as plus-size baby dolls, chemises, gowns, bustiers and corsets, teddies, hosiery and robes, garter belts, costumes, pajamas, panties, shapewear, and so on. Before choosing a lingerie style, you should always think about what suits your body shape the best, on what size you actually need, and perhaps your partner's general opinion or feeling about it. If you consider buying online, you should also check the reliability of the online store and have a good idea on how those sizes will fit your body.

While dealing with color, you do not have to be stuck choosing darker colors, for example, a white lingerie set could accentuate your curves and make you far more appealing in many cases. For many full figured, apple or pear body shapes, chiffon or satin embroidered baby dolls could be a perfect choice. Even so, you will have to figure out which color makes you feel better and matches the look you want to create for yourself. Just keep in mind that you do not have to stick to black and darker colors while making your decisions.

There are many lingerie products for plus-size women, just spend some time on the Internet searching and you will find various models and sizes.

If you are thinking of a more erotic and arousing outfit, keep in mind during your search what your partner might think or feel about lingerie. Not all men will appreciate very arousing and daring lingerie. For example, some men might be quite intimidated if following the first date you take too daring an approach. In the same scenario, some men might catalogue you as an easygoing person, while others might like it. Therefore, you should consider your partner while choosing a more daring outfit. Sometimes asking him might be a solution; in other situations, surprising him might work well. There are also many cases when keeping it simple could be the best option. A simple nightwear outfit, such as colorful flannel pajamas could work far more to your advantage and have a great effect on men.

The "taboo" chapter: How a curvy and plus-size woman could attract and win a man who likes slim women?

First, let's start by imagining your favorite fruit or dessert. In my case, that is crème caramel, while in my friend's case it is apple pie. You could go even deeper and try to imagine its shape, taste, texture, and smell. Now close your eyes for few moments and try to imagine your first bite out of it. Could you say that the picture from your mind is attractive for you? Most probably yes, because it is in your nature to find it gorgeous and succulent. Also, please notice that different people might find different desserts the most appetizing. A crème caramel is quite different from an apple pie and both are quite different from chocolate cake or ice cream. Nevertheless, any of them could be powerful enough to trigger different people.

Now the hard question comes. Will it be possible for an apple pie to outshine a crème caramel, in the case of crème caramel enthusiasts such as me? Are there cases when I will choose and prefer an apple pie instead of a crème caramel? Definitely yes, since my choices depends on many things such as:

- Availability: If I cannot find a crème caramel, I will choose an apple pie.
- Accessibility: If it is far easier for me to chose an apple pie, I will do so.
- Saturation and variation: Too much crème caramel, even visually, makes me sick.
- Timing: I am not all the time obsessed with crème caramel; there are large periods of time when I will prefer something different, such as an apple pie.
- Advertising and posture: If something else is far more intriguing to my eyes, it might have a better chance.
- Curiosity: Finding out about other sweets that I haven't tried before is appealing.

These are only a few of the possible reasons that could make me chose something else instead of my favorite dessert. Many more reasons are possible. Now, coming back to how a plus-size woman could have more success with men compared to a slim, top-model looking woman. Keep in mind that this could also work the other way around. A slim woman could also find similar ways to attract a man who normally likes curvaceous plus-size women.

As in the previous example, men have all kinds of tastes and preferences. Depending on the man, he could be more attracted by a tall or short woman, by a slim or fat woman, and so on. There were, and are, billions of men on earth, and in almost equal measure there were, and are, various preferences.

Nevertheless, how could a plus-size woman attract some men who commonly prefer a slim, top-model looking woman? Will this be possible? Yes, it should be possible in many cases. Similar to the above example, it should be possible for many plus-size women to prevail. Some key factors, which could help a plus-size woman prevail in such a case, are timing, availability, accessibility, posture, and attitude.

Availability and accessibility, especially sexual availability, are some of the most powerful tools you have as a woman. Since, to most men, availability and accessibility prevails instead of so-called beauty standards, these could be some powerful tools in the hand of a smart woman. However, playing with these is quite dangerous, since there is a thin line between using them to attract a man and creating the wrong impression. Even so, keep in mind that playing with availability and accessibility could make you more attractive for men. Try to find your own balanced, harmonious, smooth, and presentable way of handling these powerful tools.

Concluding

At various points in the past, curvaceous and plus-size women's beauty was publicly appreciated and, in many cases, preferred. You do not have centuries to wait for the mindset to change to what it was in the past. You do not have to feel bad about yourself because the mainstream media is pushing artificial commercial values. Trust in yourself. Feel confident and take care of your body in a harmonious way. Do not get your mind stuck in occasional depressive loops. Instead, focus on the long-term balance in your life. Arm yourself with a killer smile and be certain that there are many men, like us, who prefer a plus-size woman.